# Surviving American Medicine

# Surviving American Medicine

*How to Get the Right Doctor, Right Hospital,
and Right Treatment with Today's Health Care*

## Cary Presant, MD

*Foreword by Fran Drescher*

*To Gayle and Rich
Stay healthy!
Cary Presant
January, 2013*

iUniverse, Inc.
Bloomington

Surviving American Medicine
How to Get the Right Doctor, Right Hospital, and
Right Treatment with Today's Health Care

iUniverse books may be ordered through booksellers or by contacting:

iUniverse
1663 Liberty Drive
Bloomington, IN 47403
www.iuniverse.com
1-800-Authors (1-800-288-4677)

ISBN: 978-1-4759-3775-6 (sc)
ISBN: 978-1-4759-3776-3 (hc)
ISBN: 978-1-4759-3777-0 (e)

Library of Congress Control Number: 2012912456

Printed in the United States of America

iUniverse rev. date: 9/14/2012

# Praise for
# Surviving American Medicine

"As a physician experienced in giving top-notch medical care and an expert in health-care reform, Dr. Cary Presant has given us *Surviving American Medicine*, a most important, empowering book for every patient. The tips and suggestions in this outstanding book can help every person know how to get the best medical care and find answers to challenging health questions. This book enables patients to take control of their care and to know how to share decision-making with their doctors in this stressful time of health-care reform."

**Dr. Drew Pinsky**, internist and addiction specialist and host of *Dr. Drew* on HLN, *Dr. Drew's Life Changers* on national TV, and *Loveline* on national radio

---

"The knowledge we gain from reading this book is an absolute gift!"

**Fran Drescher**, writer, producer, and star of *The Nanny* and *Happily Divorced*, health-care advocate, and cancer survivor

"Providing an in-depth look at the new, consumerist health-care landscape, *Surviving American Medicine* offers a guide to put the patient in the driver's seat."

**Senator William H. Frist, MD**, cardiovascular surgeon, former majority leader of the US Senate, and health-care expert

---

"For every patient and family caregiver who is facing a serious illness, Dr. Cary Presant has written *Surviving American Medicine*, an outstanding guide for solving problems and allowing one to take control in making critical decisions. In addition, his recommendations for preventing illness and maintaining health by getting information and discussing it with the right medical providers will help people to stay healthy and live longer."

**Cindy Landon**, wife of and caregiver for actor Michael Landon, and health advocate

---

"Our health-care system delivers the highest-quality medicine in the world, but it is fragmented and complicated to access. *Surviving American Medicine*, by Cary Presant, MD, a doctor who knows how it works, is both a comprehensive and practical guide through the maze that is American medicine. His advice can save your life and bring you peace of mind. I highly recommend it to patients and doctors alike."

**Vincent T. DeVita Jr., MD**, professor at Yale Medical School, cancer expert, pioneer in oncology care, and former director of the National Cancer Institute

"*Surviving American Medicine* is a significant contribution to today's health and patient care dialogues. The distillation of lessons learned in a renowned physician-scientist's career caring for patients with cancer, its counsel is pragmatically comprehensive and philosophically sound—a vital, valuable companion for patients and families navigating through disease and illness."

**Robert Milch, MD**, expert in hospice and palliative-care, past director of Hospice Buffalo, and founding member and past president of the National Association of Hospice Physicians

---

"This 'how to' manual covers the *A* to *Z* of getting the best in health care. In easy-to-read language, with anecdotes to emphasize what can go wrong, Dr. Presant offers the consumer a handy and comprehensive guide."

**Amy Hendel**, "the HealthGal," medical and lifestyle reporter and columnist, and host of *HealthiNation.com*

---

"We applaud Dr. Presant for investing in *Surviving American Medicine*. The perspective shared and wealth of experience outlined in this resource is invaluable to patients and their loved ones as they move through their cancer journey as empowered participants."

**Kim Thiboldeaux,** President and CEO, Cancer Support Community

I dedicate this book to my family who shared me with the practice of medicine and encouraged me in this project. I love you all.

Sheila, Seth Leigh Emalyn and Rylie, Sean and Annick, Jaron Erin and Mackay, and Jaclyn

# Acknowledgments

This book has come to fruition through the support and encouragement of many individuals. I want to express my sincere thanks to all of them for what they have given me.

**My family** whose love and devotion sustained me when writing was difficult, and who inspired me to complete the project. By giving me the time to work and write, and reviewing my recommendations and the manuscript itself, you have become part of every chapter in the book. Thanks to Sheila Presant, Seth Leigh Emalyn and Rylie Presant, Sean and Annick Presant, Jaron Erin and Mackay Presant, and Jaclyn Presant.

**My extended family and close friends** who encouraged this project, shared their medical challenges with me for advice, and frankly told me of their frustrations with American medicine as they experienced it. Special thanks to Sanford and Nancy Presant, Judy and Peter Heffron, Charlotte and Louis Kimmel, Breezy and Eva Presant, Lawrence and Leslie Presant, Evelyn Hammerman, Noel and Pam Kimmel, Scott Kimmel, Scott and Katie Lassman, Jennifer and David Halperin, Heather and Kevin Scammell, Francine Linde, Nick Hanson, Eugene and Susan Spiritus, William and Barbara Sperling, Steven and Dianne Feldon, Ruedi and Karen Good, Judy and Philip Binder, Brian and Carol Joseph, and Arthur and Ricki Lane, and Alva Barozzi.

**All my patients** who told me of their successes and their frustrations. I hope I have retold your stories well enough to help other patients with their challenges.

**My role models** who have inspired me to set lofty goals, and to insist on excellence on the journey to reach those goals. I specially express my gratitude to doctors O. P. Jones, Evan Calkins, Harold Varmus, Stuart Kornfeld, Philip Majerus, Carl Moore, Vincent DeVita Jr., Emil Frei, John Mendleson, and John Baldeschwieler.

**My colleagues and medical partners** who helped me in my care of patients, who willingly shared their expertise, and who helped me to conduct my research studies to improve the care in America. Of all my colleagues, let me specially thank doctors Alex Denes, Daniel Rosenblum, Gary Ratkin, Nathan Berger, Steven Forman, Brian Carr, James Doroshow, Peter Kennedy, Charles Wiseman, Linda Bosserman, Gargi Upadhyaya, Ben Ebrahimi, Swapnil Rajurkar, Misagh Karemi, Robinson Baron, John Durant, Lawrence Baker, Charles Coltman, B. J. Kennedy, Douglas Blayney, Kirit Gala, Robert McKenna Jr., Robert Milch, Robert Moss, Lawrence Piro, and Ilene Weitz.

**My research collaborators** who have helped me develop my scientific methods and instill my passion for and rigorous critique of ideas, experiments, and results. Special thanks to Walter Wolf, Fred Valeriote, Theresa Vietti, Richard Proffitt, Carlos Perez, Geraldine Padilla, Garry Latimer, Steven Latimer, James Rutledge, Allan Hallquist, Frank Prendergast, Roy Herbst, Martin Fleisher, and Ellen Knell.

**My mentors** who taught me the skills of medicine, research, teaching, communication, and healthcare policy. I wish to especially thank doctors Arthur Serpick, Jerome Block, Julian Ambrus, Gerald Lanchantin, and William Peck.

**My fellow volunteers and coworkers** at the American Cancer Society, American Society of Clinical Oncology, Association of Community Cancer Centers, Medical Oncology Association of Southern California, American Medical Association, and Cancer Schmancer who worked beside me to help create public policy that improves the lives of Americans. I am specially grateful for having worked with Fred Mickelson, John Seffrin, Lee Mortenson, Christian Downs, Thomas Gates, Fran Drescher, Laurie Meadoff, Joseph Bailes, Ted Okon, and Mariana Lamb.

**The medical staff, nurses, physician assistants, and nurse practitioners** who have worked with me in my academic and community practices.

**The editors and advisers** at AuthorHouse and iUniverse who diligently and methodically reviewed every word, and urged me to make the critical improvements to express my experiences and suggestions more clearly and emphatically. I hope our work continues to assist people to get higher quality and more satisfying health care.

# Contents

# Foreword

*By Fran Drescher*

It was several years ago that I had the privilege of meeting Dr. Cary Presant. There we were, a couple of health-care advocates tirelessly marching on Capitol Hill in an effort to change legislation, gain funding, and improve medical care for all Americans. It was that day in the Rotunda that the bonds of our ongoing friendship were forged.

Time has not slowed us down but instead has given us greater momentum in our continuing fight to raise awareness of patients' rights. Hence my support of this most important book by Dr. Presant, whose goal of turning *patients* into *medical consumers* is of paramount importance in the twenty-first century. We are living in a time when the *business* of health care has superseded the *care* of health—a time when big-business health-insurance companies bully doctors into taking the least expensive route of diagnostic testing by threatening the doctors' contracts as preferred providers. Thus has evolved an entire generation of doctors whose philosophy is "If you hear hooves galloping, don't look for zebras, 'cause it's probably a horse." As a result, patients are being misdiagnosed and treated for the probable benign illness rather than the possible early stages of cancer. And no one knows this hard reality better than I do.

It took me two years and eight doctors to get a proper diagnosis of uterine cancer, although the symptoms I had been experiencing were classic. I swear I got in the stirrups more times than Roy Rogers! Doctor #1 said I was too young for a dilation and curettage, but I never questioned what a D&C test could have done for me because I was more thrilled to be "too young" for anything. And so it was determined that I was premenopausal, and hormone replacement therapy was prescribed. As Shakespeare said, "Therein lies the rub."

At their earliest and most curable stages, most gynecologic cancers—that is, ovarian and uterine cancers—mimic far more benign illnesses. So the woman with ovarian cancer may very well be wasting precious time being wrongly treated for irritable bowel syndrome instead. That's why 80 percent of women with ovarian cancer find out in the late stages, and 70 percent of them die of the disease. It is what killed Coretta Scott King. Similarly, uterine cancer mimics early menopause, and although it is the slowest-growing and least invasive of all the female cancers, it is the only one whose mortality rate is on the rise. It is what killed Anne Bancroft.

If we don't start taking control of our bodies, challenging our physicians, and networking to share the medical information that we know or need to know, we just might end up paying for our passivity with our lives! As it is, we Americans put more time, energy, and research into the buying, selling, and repairing of our automobiles than of our own bodies.

I know—suspecting there's something seriously wrong with you is scary. And yes, being told you have nothing to worry about comes as a relief. But don't be so accepting of a first opinion. When you consider the way our health-care system works, with its high rate of improper treatment and late-stage cancer diagnoses, taking one doctor's word for anything is, at the very least, stupid—and at the very worst, suicidal.

I promise you I would not be here today were it not for my persistence in getting second opinions. Doctors are not gods. They're human beings with their own lives and problems. When the doctor calls to tell you that you have cancer, at the end of the day he goes home to eat dinner with his family while you go home to eat your heart out with yours. You owe it to yourself and your loved ones not to become an ostrich when faced with poor health. At that moment more than any, you must become a brave soldier, ready for combat. Rise to the challenge and meet your obstacle head-on, with relentless perseverance.

Gather your allies; never go to any appointments alone. Bring along a list of questions, as well as a pen and paper to write down the answers. Ask to have things spelled out so that you can research them yourself later. And never let a busy doctor rush you or intimidate you. Treat your appointment as you would any business transaction. A patient is a customer, and the customer is always right!

In your search for better health, consider your lifestyle as well. All too often doctors treat the symptoms of an illness when both doctor and patient should be focused on preventing the illness through changes to lifestyle and nutrition. To this end, I urge you to buy organic whenever possible. (Nowadays, even Walmart sells organic products, so the option is available to most consumers.) And eat predominantly whole foods, rather than processed. First rule of thumb: if a food looks like its original form, it's a whole food. It goes without saying that fruits and vegetables doused with pesticides simply can't be good for us.

As a nation we are far too dependent on prescription drugs as the answer to all our medical ailments—and that should come as no surprise when pharmaceutical companies make huge profits by targeting physicians and patients with drug promotions and incentives. Where is the incentive to eat healthier foods, such as brown rice, rather than relying on food extracts and nutritional supplements? Learn the tests available for the cancers that could affect you; the cancer-screening test you need may not even be on the menu at your doctor's office.

During my recovery, not one doctor discussed nutrition with me. This conversation only occurred when I made an appointment with an acupuncturist because I wasn't feeling well after my surgery. It was he who enlightened me about how my diet has a direct influence on how I feel.

Experience has convinced me that it is imperative that we take responsibility for our own health. We must change the way we think, eat, and live—it is, literally, a matter of life and death. And reading Dr. Presant's book is a great first step. Presant is an appropriate name for our author, because the knowledge we gain from reading this book is an absolute gift!

*Fran Drescher*

# Introduction

## Medicine Today: What's It All About?

Health-care reform isn't just political rhetoric: it's a reality. It's happening every day. And for you it means new ways of getting your medical care. The modernization of the insurance industry is resulting in broad changes to health-care coverage and benefits, and many individuals are losing their employer-provided health insurance. At the same time, medical costs have dramatically increased. Because of a shortage of doctors, medical care frequently falls to nurse practitioners or physicians' assistants. Higher costs in the medical office are resulting in fewer staff, less attention to patients, shorter visits, and a reduced focus on preventing disease and following health-care guidelines. In order to stave off financial losses, hospitals are reducing staff and using hospitalists in place of patients' own physicians; the result is lower patient satisfaction, less attentive care, and more medical errors. And because insurance companies insist on shortened hospital stays, hospitalists are transferring more patients into skilled nursing facilities and rehabilitation centers. Costs have risen dramatically at the pharmaceutical level too, as new medications are anywhere from ten to one thousand times more expensive than old standards, overburdening family budgets.

So virtually every American is aware that we are experiencing dramatic changes in the delivery of health care and the insurance programs that pay for it. Through the 2010 Patient Protection and Affordable Care Act, updates to Medicare and its funding, and the American Reinvestment and Recovery Act, the federal government has mandated revised insurance programs, changes in health-care delivery, improved electronic health records, and medical information protections for all Americans. Legislation and regulation at the state level is further affecting the care you receive and how your doctors (and their practices) treat you and talk to you. With all the new regulations, new technologies, new drugs, and new types of surgery, change has become incessant. Patients feel lost, unable to control or improve the mess of dealing with their health and their conditions. And when a personal health crisis occurs, making the right decisions seems impossible.

The fact is, times have changed, and they're not changing back. In today's American health-care landscape, you are now in charge of your own well-being. You are steering the boat, so to speak. And to do so efficiently and well, you need to know how to navigate the waters.

In the old paradigm of medical care, you trusted the doctor (who was completely committed to your well-being) and the hospital (which was well-staffed and compassionate enough to keep you in your bed until you really felt well) to make all the best decisions for you. And they did just that. Your insurance company wouldn't cancel your policy, and it paid most of your bills, which were affordable.

In the contemporary paradigm, there are much better tests, treatments, and results; you live longer; and many diseases are prevented, or they are delayed in onset and well-controlled. Those are remarkable benefits. But medicine has become astronomically expensive, and insurance frequently denies payments for the new, promising treatments you've been hearing about in the media. Now you have more responsibility to make shared decisions with physicians (or their nurse practitioners), who have little time to explain all the information you need to make those decisions. You have less time to ask questions, while the doctor spends more time with technology—reading reports, updating your electronic health record, reviewing test results, and ordering your complex treatment plan, which will be sent digitally to the nurses, hospital, insurance provider, and consultants. The good news is that medicine is better. The bad news is it's tougher for you to get good medical care and feel confident about it.

That's what this book is designed to do—to help you make choices about your health care so you will feel confident that you're getting the best treatment possible. You'll learn what goes on behind the doors of the hospitals and insurance companies so you will know how to get the best doctors, how to argue false charges on your bills, how to pick the best insurance coverage, and how to ensure that at the end of the day, you're in control—not simply being manipulated by giant corporations, whether they are insurance companies, hospitals, physician networks, health-maintenance organizations, or accountable-care organizations.

If you have no health insurance, start with section 4, "Insuring and Financing Your Health Care," to find advice on insurance programs and dealing with claims. If you have insurance but no primary-care physician, start with section 1, "Getting the Right Health Plan," where you will find tips on retaining and communicating with doctors. If you have developed an illness or condition, you will find recommendations in section 2, "Dealing with Disease and Serious Illness," that can help you overcome your challenges. Section 3, "Caring for Others," includes advice on being a caregiver/advocate for family or friends (the young, the elderly, and the infirmed) as well as advice on using hospitals.

Just to let you know, I will refer you to specific organizations and their websites for supportive information, and the web addresses I provide were current when I wrote *Surviving American Medicine*. But websites can change, so if an address listed here is no longer current, look up the organization using a search engine like Google, and you will get the new address.

I hope you won't need to use every chapter in this book. If you're lucky, you already have good health insurance—insurance that covers both your current health issues and your preventive health care, and that makes the correct decisions about approving the care you need—preparing you for the acute accidents, serious diseases, and chronic ailments that appear as you grow older. And if you've been fortunate, you already have an excellent physician who is up-to-date, caring, and aggressive about preventing the serious, life-threatening illnesses that life brings.

But even if you have all that, chances are something will change in the future. Your insurance company may make changes that omit some medical services it previously covered. Or your trusted doctor might retire or get ill, fail to keep up with medical advances, or join a practice plan that changes how much he cares about you. As the health-care landscape has shifted, more physicians have been selling their practices to hospitals, retiring early, or joining larger clinics or networks. And with each of these changes, the doctor is expected to meet new objectives, achieve different goals, and/or perform at higher productivity standards, none of which is likely to benefit the patients.

This book will start you on the process of taking control of these issues, empowering you to work with your team of doctors, nurses, hospitals, and even insurance companies to maintain your health and prolong your life. It is designed to give you access to the insider tips I've garnered from my forty years as a physician, professor, administrator, and researcher. Together we will look at the shortcomings of today's medical system, as viewed through the true stories and frustrations that my patients, my friends, and even my doctor colleagues have shared with me. Learn from their mistakes. Do what they didn't. Keep pushing where they stopped. You'll probably live longer as a result.

## Inside Your Doctor's Head

Despite all the problems with health care, on many levels we're still living in the best of times. American life expectancy has dramatically increased in the past hundred years. In 1900, the average life expectancy was only 49.2 years (*Congressional Research Service Report*, Aug. 16, 2006). By 2010, it had increased to 78.7 years (*Centers for Disease Control National Vital Statistics Report for 2010*, Jan. 11, 2012). We expect to see that number top 80 years soon.

What accounts for this increase? Well, diet, exercise, and healthier food account for some of it, but without a doubt the major factor is advances in health care. New treatments are emerging every day, even for the worst diseases. Complex, advanced surgeries are becoming commonplace. Organ transplants are everyday procedures. New drugs have been developed to control hypertension, cardiovascular disease, Alzheimer's disease, cancer, blood diseases, liver disease, and infections. Scientists now know the human genetic code, and soon they will be using synthetic genes or gene-targeted drugs to cure many medical conditions. And to serve it all up, we've developed a comprehensive health-care delivery system, which can bring these advances to patients in almost any community.

But for all our advances, this is also a time of crisis in American medicine. The quality of medical care in America is not uniform. While some patients are satisfied with their health and their doctors, many others complain about the lack of good medical care and poor results: continued symptoms, worsening illnesses, limited access to tests, inadequate information, and a general lack of confidence in the system.

But an even bigger problem is the inconsistency of insurance coverage. Some patients have health plans that allow them to have standard and state-of-the-art treatments, while others either lack insurance altogether or have insurance companies that seem to do nothing but obstruct their care. How can this inequity in quality medical care occur here, in the most advanced nation in the world?

To put it simply, the system is stressed. Contemporary medicine is characterized by the problems of uninsured or underinsured patients; inconsistent care which often doesn't meet national quality guidelines; lack of disease prevention; care that is too expensive (and becomes more so every year); less attention by doctors and nurses; and lack of access for many patients. Our attempts to solve these chronic problems change the health-care landscape every year.

Knowing these problems and understanding the impact of the changes on your personal care can help you get the attention you need when you need it. And by doing some research on your own, you can find the answers you need more quickly. Assume that your care will change, and take advantage of the solutions that will keep you prepared. Then you'll be empowered to survive the conditions and changes which are optimistically called "health-care reform."

## Why I Wrote This Book

There's a phrase that seems to permeate every advertisement we see or read: "Ask your doctor about …" It seems to be the media's first advice, whether the subject is fatigue, weight loss, depression, erectile dysfunction, heart disease, cancer, Alzheimer's, or any other medical condition, large or small.

This is a sign that *you* are now in control of your own health care. Gone are the days when you could rely on your doctor to tell you about all the medical options that are out there. Now it's up to you to pick up the slack.

Good luck. To take charge of your health care and make smart decisions, you need more information and advice—which usually your doctor no longer has the time to provide. You are mostly on your own! That's why I wrote this book, to give you information that will guide you in those decisions. These tips will help you identify the issues that are important for your care and teach you how to discuss them successfully with your doctors and nurses.

At every party, community meeting, and dinner I attend, I get questions from people seeking more advice on a health-care problem. "My insurance is changing. What plan should I pick?" "I can't stand my doctor's attitude. Who can you suggest?" "My medicines aren't working. What should I do?" "My husband's health is failing. Where can I go for help?" My passion is helping patients like these take charge of their health so that, together with their physicians, they can make the best decisions about their own care.

*Surviving American Medicine* will help you and your family with perplexing problems and difficult decisions as I share what I've learned from years of experience assisting patients, family, and friends. Your life will be simpler and healthier as a result.

In *Surviving American Medicine*, I have included my patients' compelling stories. Except for Michael Landon, I have changed the name of each patient for confidentiality. To help you read the text more easily, I have varied the use of male and female pronouns ("he" or "she") in describing physicians, patients, nurses, nurse practitioners and health advocates.

Section 1:
# Getting the
# Right Health Plan

# Chapter 1

# Selecting a Primary-Care Physician: How to Find a "Keeper"

Melanie had developed a cough, and she was referred by her primary physician, Dr. Jones, to a lung specialist who performed a bronchoscopy. Unfortunately, the news was bad: lung cancer. The specialist did not check back with Dr. Jones; instead he directly referred Melanie to an oncologist he knew. Melanie waited several days before the oncologist's office called to tell her she would have to wait another two weeks for her appointment. At her wit's end with anxiety, Melanie called Dr. Jones to see if there was a faster way to get her lifesaving treatments started. Similarly frustrated, Dr. Jones recommended a different oncologist, one she would use for someone in her own family if cancer were diagnosed. In fact, Dr. Jones took it a step further and had her staff call the new oncologist and make an emergency appointment. Within two days, Melanie was seen and treated. Her cancer was cured.

Your choice of primary-care physician (and of any specialist, for that matter) will determine whether you survive as long and as well as you can. As the one person who keeps you well, gives you the vaccinations you need, helps you improve your health habits, evaluates and treats your symptoms when you first have them, and evaluates your risk of future illness and advises you how to prevent it, your primary-care physician is your first key to wellness and health. So it's critical that you find the best doctor for you—a "keeper."

In fact, one of the most common questions people ask me is, "How can I find a good doctor?" Too often this is a frustrating process, and people are left to rely on a physician hotline or a hospital locator. Granted, these services are better than nothing, but usually they don't attract the top docs.

As in my patient Melanie's true story, the best way to set up a medical-care team is to start at its center, with the primary-care physician: a family practitioner, internist, gynecologist, or pediatrician. These doctors are your first line of defense, the front line of clinicians who will take care of colds, symptoms, vaccinations, checkups, and other common complaints. They're also your key to finding good specialists should the need arise.

The good news is that, in my experience, more than 70 percent of patients like and trust their primary-care physicians. They've been lucky enough to find doctors who are up-to-date on the newest therapies, responsive, and genuinely caring.

But then there are the other 30 percent. What are they to do?

The sad fact is that most of them remain with the doctors they hate, paralyzed by the thought of hunting down a new physician, worried that maybe *they* are the ones with the problem, not the doctor.

If you're in that group, don't worry. The fact is, even if your doctor is a good clinician, and even if your doctor is world-famous, if the doctor makes you feel uncomfortable, that doctor is not the right one for you.

## Finding Your Perfect Doctor

Different people want different types of doctors. Some want a doctor to be direct and say, "This is what you have to do—no questions!" Others want the doctor to give them all the options, from *A* to *Z*, so they can make an informed choice.

Regardless, there are a few things everyone should look for in a physician, whether he or she is a primary-care physician or a specialist:

**Intelligence:**

Did the doctor attend a well-recognized college and medical school?

Does the doctor explain complex plans or conditions logically and explain the rationale for any tests or treatments?

Does the doctor answer your questions authoritatively?

**Up-to-date knowledge:**

Does your doctor recommend the most current treatments, not ones that have been used for years?

When you ask about a new treatment you've heard or read about, is the doctor already knowledgeable about it?

Does your doctor give you the latest findings from a recent medical meeting or journal?

When you ask about prevention or genetics, does your doctor have an answer, and does that answer include the words *new* or *current*?

**Willingness to make a judgment or commitment:**

When you have new problems or concerns, does the doctor order tests or just say, "We'll see what happens"?

Does the doctor stand up for you when your insurance company or HMO requires authorization or denies coverage?

**Solid knowledge base:**

There are national guidelines for disease prevention, symptom evaluation, and treatment. A good doctor is familiar with these and uses them to help diagnose you quickly and completely.

**Good bedside manner:**

You should be able to talk to your doctor easily and feel that he or she is listening to you. Also, your doctor should explain things clearly and completely and ask if you have any questions.

**A kind office staff:**

These are the first people you will have to deal with at a doctor's office, and they should treat you with respect and dignity.

**Compassion:**

You should always feel that your doctor cares about you and is on your side, no matter what. If you become ill, your doctor is your partner in the trenches.

## The Search

Okay, so now you know what to look for in a doctor. The next question is, how do you find it? Here are some tips.

- **Step 1: Ask family, friends, and neighbors for their recommendations.** We tend to trust the advice of friends and relatives, and their advice can be very detailed. Most important, they really enjoy telling you all the good and bad points of their interactions with their physician. Usually they will answer all your questions about the doctor: what she (or he) is like, whether she smiles, how easy it is to understand her, whether she takes the time to answer all your questions, whether she makes sense when speaking. But always ask *why* they like the doctor, since their preferences may be based only on personality. You may not be looking for the same qualities, so the doctor who's best for them may not be the best one for you! Above all, don't be afraid to ask around about a doctor. The more people you ask, the more you'll find out, and the better you'll know if that doctor is a good physician, not just a nice person.

- **Step 2: Ask your best source of information: your prior doctor.** Most people already have had a primary-care physician, either a family practitioner or an internist. If you need a new primary-care physician or a specialist, your primary doctor can usually suggest a good one. Ask your referring doctor these important questions:
  - How good is the doctor? (As good as you? As good as the doctors at any university? The best in the area?)
  - What is the doctor's commitment to his or her patients?
  - How well does the doctor communicate with patients?
  - How is the doctor's bedside manner?
  - Is the doctor prompt?
  - Does the doctor call the referring physician right away to discuss all findings, diagnoses, and therapies?
  - How well do the doctor's patients typically do?
  - And the very best question to ask a referring doctor: "Would you personally go to this doctor or send your family to him?"
  - If you've just moved to a new area or you've switched health plans (with a new list of panel physicians), ask your previous doctor about any physicians he might know in your new community or in your new health plan. He will usually have the broadest experience with specialists and consultants and can give you the most insightful evaluation.

- **Step 3: Ask doctors you know socially.** Do you have a doctor friend—maybe through a club, church, or PTA? Does a doctor live in your neighborhood? If not, maybe someone in your family or a close friend knows a doctor she could call on your behalf. If so, ask that doctor to recommend a physician who offers high-quality care appropriate for you. And remember, never be afraid to ask, "Would you go to this doctor for your own care—and if so, why?" I know most people hesitate to ask for this sort of advice, but you should know that most doctors love being asked to recommend a colleague. You're letting the doctor know that you value his advice and opinion.

- **Step 4: Rely on nurses as an important source of information.** If a nurse works in a hospital or in an office where you are considering getting care, she knows the reputation of the hospitals and physicians based on personal critical experience. Nurses observe patient care firsthand. They are the first to praise physicians who give excellent care, and they are the first to warn you about physicians who don't. Once again, be sure to ask as many questions as possible about why they would or would not recommend a particular doctor.

- **Step 5: Read the lists of "best" doctors in your city.** These lists can be found in magazines, books, or newspapers, and most of them are based on physician recommendations, like those found in the books *Best Doctors in America* and *America's Top Doctors*. Also check magazines with articles like "The Best Doctors in Your City." Check with your local library for newspapers or magazines, or look for a list online. But for any doctor listed, always check out other sources too. Even a highly regarded doctor might have a particular practice style which may not appeal to you. (For example, some doctors see patients only after a trainee has completed an initial evaluation; others may use physicians' assistants.) Check the website of Castle Connolly (CastleConnolly.com) to see a partial list from *America's Top Doctors*. Other commonly used sites which list and describe doctors are HealthGrades.com, AngiesList.com, Vitals.com, and AMD-ASSN.org/aps/amagh.htm, the website of the American Medical Association. Government sources include the National Institutes of Health and its resource library, Medline, which offers a complete list of physicians at NIM.NIH.gov/medlineplus/directories.html. I strongly suggest using all these sites to get as much information as possible about any doctor you are interested in using. More information means a better decision.

- **Step 6: Use patient support groups for trustworthy recommendations.** If you've got a chronic condition or a serious illness, you may find patient support groups (like the American Cancer Society or the Cancer Support Community) at your local hospital[1] or even on the Internet. Always try to find a local chapter so that you can talk face-to-face with other patients. They are usually very honest about what they think of their care.

- **Step 7: Use your insurance company's list.** If you have a health plan (including private insurance, a PPO, or an HMO), the insurance company can provide you with a list of physicians with whom they contract. Get this list and review which doctors are in your area or are contracted with your independent practice association (IPA). If you have questions, call the insurance carrier. Just remember that this list does not discriminate or delineate good doctors from bad. That's up to you to find out.

- **Step 8: Once you have identified a good candidate, check the physician out.** First, go to the computer and "Google" the doctor. If you don't know how, ask a friend, neighbor, or librarian to help you—it's easy. All the websites and articles in which the doctor's name is mentioned will pop up, and you can read them. Most doctors have a website listing all their credentials. But if the doctor in question has no website—and that is not a good sign, since most physicians who care about their practice and their patients will have one, except for some older doctors—then just call the office and ask the secretary for the doctor's curriculum vitae (commonly called the "CV"). That's the doctor's biography, and every office has one; hospitals require it when a physician applies for staff privileges, and insurance companies need it to grant malpractice insurance or a contract. If your doctor won't give you a copy of his CV, be skeptical. (What else might the doctor not let you see?) The technical terms in the CV might be confusing, but most of the credentials are easily understood as follows:

---

1    To find a support group, call your local hospital and ask to talk to the nursing department or the department of community education. They will tell you if the hospital has such a support group or can refer you to one in the community. If they can't suggest one, call a larger hospital in a nearby community or a tertiary-care teaching hospital in your city and ask for the same departments.

- **Licensure and training:** Where a doctor has trained is a good indication of the quality of her knowledge and of the medical care you will receive. Foreign medical schools are generally regarded as inferior to American ones. And the best American schools are well-known: Harvard, Yale, Columbia, Cornell, Johns Hopkins, Stanford, UCLA.
- **Board certifications:** These reflect the passing of tests based upon total medical knowledge. You should only use a doctor with board certification in primary care (family practice, internal medicine, obstetrics/gynecology) or in the specialty relevant to the care you need.
- **Honors and awards:** Professional accolades show that a doctor's colleagues consider his knowledge or work to be remarkable and above average.
- **Publications:** A doctor's published work reflects additional knowledge, intelligence, and achievement, and it offers clues to whether the doctor is an expert in your conditions or illnesses. You should note carefully if the doctor has published papers or given lectures about your ailment, since such experience usually means that the doctor is current in his understanding of recent advances or has access to the latest treatments, including clinical trials.
- **Professional organizations:** Membership in professional organizations indicates how well the physician keeps up with advances in the field.

- **Step 9: Check to see if the doctor has been in trouble.** You can get a report from the state licensing board about a doctor's malpractice experience. (See appendix 4 for a list of state medical boards and their phone numbers.) The board can tell you if the doctor has been placed on probation or censured, the history of any malpractice suits, if his hospital privileges have ever been revoked, or if his license has ever been cancelled.

- **Step 10: Don't use a "find a doctor" service.** Unfortunately, these services are everywhere you look, and they'll list anyone who will write them a check. The lists are not dependent on quality or credentials—just on who will pay them for patient referrals. Similarly, be wary of the recommendations of hospital referral offices. They simply rotate through the medical staff; they cannot exclude doctors based on poor performance or recommend them based on good service. That being said, if you have no other outlets, you can start with these lists, as long as you do your own research and check out the doctors they recommend before you see them. If they don't check out, ask for more names and keep looking until you find someone you like.

- **Step 11: Work to get an appointment with a physician you've chosen.** Here's a major roadblock a lot of patients run into: you find someone you like, but when you call for an appointment you're told her schedule is too full and she's not taking new patients. However, if you have any personal contact with the doctor through a social organization or friend, or if you have a personal referral or recommendation from one of her friends, patients, or colleagues, that might be enough for her to make an exception. Be sure to tell the office staff you have a *personal* connection when you call for an appointment. If necessary, ask another doctor you know to make the call to request an appointment.

- **Step 12: If you don't have a personal connection, think "six degrees."** The old adage that "everyone is connected to everyone else by at most six degrees of separation" can be a valuable tool when it comes to personal referrals. The unspoken truth is that when you use someone's name as a referral, doctors rarely check to see how well you know that person. If a doctor you like can't take you, ask his office staff to recommend another doctor they like. Research that doctor, and if you like what you see, use the previous doctor's office as a referral source when you call to make the appointment. If necessary, ask a friend for the name of a physician he trusts. Then can call that doctor's office to get the name of a specialist that doctor uses.

- **Step 13: Don't be intimidated.** A lot of people clam up when they talk to doctors. They feel that they are in a realm they don't understand, and so they automatically assume a passive position—afraid to ask questions when they're confused, or to push a little when they need something. Don't fall into this trap. I'm not suggesting that you be rude—on the contrary, be as nice and polite as you possibly can—but when you're told no, don't just hang up or walk away. Ask for a referral to someone else.

It often helps to have your notes in front of you when you ask for an appointment, so you are less intimidated by the call. And if the receptionist declines your request, always ask to talk to the office manager or the doctor for a final decision.

When Terry switched to an HMO, for example, her prior primary-care doctor was not on the HMO's three-hundred-page list of contracted doctors. When a doctor looked through the list and suggested Dr. Gates, Terry called Dr. Gates, but his nurse said they couldn't take any new patients, even those with personal connections. A little angry, Terry pushed further, asking Dr. Gates's staff if they could possibly recommend another doctor, and they came up with a couple of names, one of whom matched Terry's HMO provider list. She did some research online and decided she liked the doctor's credentials, so she found a hospital where he had attending privileges and talked to a nurse there, just to get a second opinion. Satisfied that she had found someone good, Terry called and made an appointment. In her conversation with the office staff, she was careful to say, "I was referred to you by Dr. Gates." (Not a lie—technically, she was.) Two weeks later, Terry had made appointments for her entire family. They've been with the same doctor for three years now and are completely satisfied with their care. By persevering and doing your homework, as Terry did, you can find a good doctor too.

## Concierge and VIP Medical Services

There's a new twist to finding a good primary doctor, and it's a bit more expensive. Certain practices are now offering a special service called "concierge medicine" or "retainer medicine," which provides you more face-to-face time with the doctor, more preventive services, and shorter waits in return for a monthly or yearly fee. In exchange for an initial sign-up cost of $1,500 to $30,000 plus an annual fee of $1,000 to $25,000, these VIP practices also give you faster access to doctors by phone, not only during office hours but also on weekends or holidays. These services represent added costs beyond those of maintaining your standard insurance, which you should not discontinue. The price range for these services varies widely depending on the area where you live and the prestige of the physician (which does not always relate to the quality of his work, but more to what he feels he is worth). Most practices tend toward the lower cost range.

Is access to a more responsive doctor worth this added fee? That's up to you. For some people, it's valuable to have someone else personally help you select a consultant or get an appointment with a preferred specialist. They'll gladly pay for shorter wait times, more comprehensive screening, more frequent checkups, and the feeling of security and special care that such concierge physician services can provide.

Keep in mind, however, that no one is guaranteeing the quality of the services you receive. Just because a doctor commits to giving you VIP-type service, that does not mean that she is a top-notch doctor or that you will like the type of care and bedside manner she'll provide. Before signing up with such a service, be sure to get recommendations from others who have used it, and get a complete list of the available doctors. And keep in mind that if you have already chosen a good doctor (by using the process outlined above), you may have no need for VIP or concierge service.

I've seen patients become very stressed when their physician suddenly decides to convert to concierge service, mandating that after a certain date, all patients will have to pay the special fee to continue to be a patient, or else they must find another doctor. If that happens to you, what should you do then? Consider whether you want to pay the extra fee. If you don't, start looking for another doctor using the steps outlined above. You can even ask your current doctor whom to select; doctors who make this switch usually already have another doctor in mind who does not charge the concierge fee.

*Surviving American Medicine* is designed to help you to find good physicians so you can avoid having to pay for concierge services. You should feel empowered to do the research and get the care you need within the parameters of the insurance plan you have selected and paid for.

The key point to remember is that whether you do it yourself or you pay someone else to do it, the homework must be done if you want to make an informed decision about who's administering your medical care.

## Tips

- Commit yourself to finding a good primary-care physician so you can stay well, prevent disease, and check out symptoms as soon as they occur.
- Know the characteristics you are looking for in a doctor—beyond just a nice personality.
- Follow the thirteen steps described above.
- Check out any doctor before you make an appointment.
- If an appointment isn't immediately available, work to get one anyway.

## Contemporary Medicine and Finding a Doctor

Whether dramatic changes occur as part of legislated health-care reform or the system just continues to slowly change with time, you will always need to find good doctors as your primary-care physician and specialists. And that will get trickier, since many doctors might not be contracted with your health-insurance plan (HMO, PPO, IPA, ACO, Medicare, or Medicaid). Fewer doctors in a plan means more shopping to find your doctor.

By using the suggestions I've listed above, you will be able to get the right doctor for you—which brings us to the next topic.

# Chapter 2

# Your First Physician Visit

If you are about to see a new physician, you need to be prepared. The suggestions in this chapter will help you make that experience a good one, giving you confidence and facilitating a strong doctor-patient relationship.

Initially, you'll have two tasks: first to get your new doctor's thoughts on keeping you well, the state of your health, and evaluation of any worrisome symptoms; and second to figure out if he is someone you can trust. Since you might be a little uncomfortable and even a little scared (although you shouldn't be, and *Surviving American Medicine* will help you become more self-assured), you probably don't envision this initial visit as an opportunity to run your physician through a game of twenty questions. But the fact is, this is *exactly* the time to do just that. You will never get as much attention from your physician as you will during this first visit. And the more organized you are in asking all the important questions, the better you can discern if this is the right doctor for you. This will be your confidence-building time. Consider bringing a family member or friend with you to help you evaluate the doctor, remember his answers, and remind you to ask him all your questions.

## First Impressions

Before you've even talked to the doctor or staff, you can begin evaluating how well his office might work for you. The clues are all sitting right there in the waiting room. Consider the following:

- Is the office neat and clean?
- Does the office staff help you complete all the necessary forms and get the proper authorizations? State and federal laws require a barrage of paperwork, so do not be frightened by how thick the packet is. The staff should be happy to assist you in filling the forms out.
- Does the office pay prompt attention to you and apologize for any delay?
- Are the other patients happy with the care they receive there? Don't be afraid to ask; the more you talk with other patients, the more of an inside scoop you will get.
- What does the office expect you to do while you're waiting? Is there medical information available? Are the magazines recent? Are there enough seats for everyone? How long have others been waiting?

## Talking with the Doctor's Staff

If you're going to like a doctor, you have to like his staff, because they are your contact point. So prepare a list of questions to evaluate them, as well. Consider the following:

- Is there enough staff to handle all the patients at the desk and in the exam rooms?
- Is the staff organized—do they have your information, your test results, and your chart available? Do they seem concerned about you?
- What is their opinion of the doctor? Is he usually on time? Will he spend extra time with you if necessary? Will he let you take notes or record the conversation? Will he write notes for you about your treatment plan? Will you be able to read his report about your visit? Ask the receptionist and the office

manager these questions, and then ask to get a copy of the doctor's visit report when you leave the office. (If he dictates the report or completes it later, ask the staff to send you a copy when it is completed).

## Breaking the Ice with the Doctor: Your Introduction

Once you've gotten past the office staff and decided you like them, it's time for the main event—meeting your physician.

Where do you begin? For starters, let the doctor know who or what brought you to the office (another doctor's recommendation or another satisfied patient). Let the doctor know if the word on the street about his office is good. Then explain your goals—your health history and what issues concern you.

Think of this as any other business meeting—a consultation with a potential new business partner, a colleague at work, or a job applicant. The doctor is, after all, going to be a valuable new asset to your team. As you talk, consider the doctor's demeanor:

- Does the doctor shake hands with you, maintain eye contact, and perhaps give you a friendly touch or hug?
- When writing in the chart or typing an electronic note, does the doctor look up and actually see how you are responding?
- Does the doctor know what's in your chart, or does he constantly have to keep checking it?
- Can you understand the doctor's questions? Does he respond to yours?
- Does the doctor seem to view you comprehensively (he's concerned about your health and disease prevention, not just about your symptom or biggest problem)? Is he honest, open, interested, trustworthy, personable, conversational, and concerned about you as an individual, not just a person with an ailment?
- Do you feel comfortable and at ease with the doctor, or tense and fearful?

## What Do You Ask, and How Do You Ask It?

Most people are afraid of confronting their doctor. In fact, many are more fearful of the doctor than of the illness itself. This is understandable. The reality is that most people don't have any contact with the medical world *until* they are sick. To make matters worse, many physicians are hurried and stressed and don't have the extra time to spend with new patients. So an office visit can feel like you're walking into someone else's whirlwind.

But getting the best care requires a lot of conversation and interaction. This is not the time to be quiet and submissive. So remember: *make a list of all your questions ahead of time.* (Even doctors do this when visiting their own physicians.) If you're intimidated, have a friend or relative come with you and ask the questions for you. And if a doctor gets annoyed at reasonable questions, take that as a sign you should find another doctor. You're looking for a sense of mutual trust and respect here.

If you're stuck on where to begin the conversation, consider the following examples.

General questions:

- How healthy am I? Are there conditions that I am developing? (Expect a detailed answer.)
- What is my risk of common illnesses, like heart disease, cancer, lung or kidney disease, or bone problems? What can I do to prevent or delay them? (Expect an answer regarding each disease and specifics about nutrition, diet, medications, and lifestyle changes.)
- What routine tests and screening procedures do I need? (Expect descriptions of cholesterol, glucose, and kidney function tests, mammograms, carotid ultrasounds, PSAs, colonoscopies, Pap smears, HPV screenings, or any other applicable tests.)
- Will you talk about nutrition, diet, exercise, and complementary therapies? (Expect answers regarding each subject.)
- How do you keep up with advances in medicine? (Expect a description of the meetings and lectures the doctor attends and journals he reads.)

- How do I see copies of my chart and my reports, and can I get copies of your notes and records from any consultations, laboratory tests, or X-rays? Do you use electronic health records, and can I get a copy of my note each time I see you? Will you tell me what types of screening procedures I need for all the different diseases? How do you or your nurses keep track of what vaccinations I need? Do you ever make house calls? If I were sick and could not come in, where would you ask me to go? (Expect a description of how you get copies of your record and how the doctor gets reminders of things you need. Most doctors don't make house calls, but be impressed if he does.)
- If I have a problem, how difficult would it be for me to reach you? Who will answer my questions on the phone? Do you use nurse practitioners or physicians' assistants in your office, and how do you decide who sees me when I'm sick? Who covers for you when you are on vacation or at a medical meeting? How would they know my case history should the need arise? Would you be available to discuss my case with the covering physician, even if you were out of town? (Expect the doctor to have a good coverage system and responsive communication procedures.)

Questions about your medical condition or symptoms:

- What's wrong with me, and how do you propose treating me? Will you write down exactly what you want me to do? (Expect clear answers and written lists if you need them.)
- Do you have other patients with my disease? How did they do? Can I talk to anyone with a similar condition? (You should be able to speak with other patients if they agree.)
- What are the complications of the treatment you're recommending? Are these complications very likely to occur? How severe will they be? Will they be permanent? (Expect details and percentages, not generalities.)
- What drugs or procedures will be necessary? Do they have side effects? What is their success rate? (Expect an understandable plan with few side effects and a high success rate—over 90 percent.)

Questions about surgery, if applicable:

- How many of these specific operations did you do last year? What is your success rate? What is your complication rate? Is there a death rate from the operation? If there were a complication, when would you tell my family and me? (Expect the doctor to have performed at least five procedures per year with a complication rate under 5 percent and a mortality rate under 1 percent.)
- Is there any alternative to the surgery? (Expect clear descriptions of alternative types of surgery and the typical success of nonsurgical management.)
- Is the diagnosis certain, or is it possible something else could be wrong? Do I need a second opinion on the diagnosis, the X-rays, or the biopsy results? (Expect the doctor to be willing to get a second opinion on the diagnostic tests or biopsies, and to have high confidence that his diagnosis is correct.)
- If I require surgery, do I need it right away, or can it be delayed? (Expect a description of the risk of waiting.)
- Do I have any other illnesses or conditions, or am I taking any medicine that could raise my risk of complications from this surgery? (Expect the doctor to be aware of all your other illnesses and medications and to describe all possible complications and their rates.)
- What tests do I need before any surgery to be certain that it is actually necessary and that I will have no risk of complications? (Your doctor or nurse should have given you a complete list of preoperative tests, including blood tests and chest X-rays, and an EKG if there is any suspicion of heart disease.)
- Which hospital would you want me to go to and why? What is the complication rate there? What is the infection rate? What is the hospital's rate of severe antibiotic-resistant infections (MRSA or VRE)? (Expect a comparison of potential hospitals. An acceptable resistant infection rate is less than 5 percent.)

Be specific with your questions, write them down ahead of time, and don't be afraid to ask whatever's on your mind. Use this visit to learn about your ailment and what causes it, why you suffer from your symptoms, and what you can do about them. Then judge the doctor's responses accordingly.

A patient of mine summed it up like this: "You just need to find a doctor who makes it perfectly clear—not too technical, not too complex. You just have to be able to understand what's wrong." *A doctor who can't make it "perfectly clear" is not the right doctor for you.*

## Tips

- Be prepared with questions you need to ask the doctor. Make sure they're written down so you do not forget any.
- Bring a family member or friend to help you.
- Observe the staff closely and pay attention to the appearance of the office.
- Ask all your questions, listen carefully, and then ask follow-up questions.
- At the end of the visit, evaluate how the doctor and the office appeared to you and whether the doctor seems right for you.

## Today's Medicine and Your First Visit

All the changes in health-care reform will mean less time at each doctor visit, including the first one. To make matters worse, any visit you have may be with a "mid-level provider"—that is, a nurse practitioner or physician's assistant. (See the chapter on these important players on your health-care team.) So you must have your questions thought out and written down in advance, and if you are overwhelmed by the stress and worry of the visit, have a patient advocate (a family member or friend) with you to ask the questions for you. Be sure someone (you or your advocate) writes down the doctor's answers or records them on a smart phone or a little tape recorder (really cheap and really helpful). So bring paper, pencil, and/or pen. *If the physician, nurse practitioner, or physician's assistant does not answer all your questions to your understanding, this may not be the right doctor for you.*

# Chapter 3

# Evaluating Your Physician

## The Doctor's Scorecard

If you're not familiar with the medical world, it can be difficult to know exactly what you should be able to expect from your doctor. What follows is a short list of the desirable characteristics for your health-care provider—a scorecard by which you can measure your doctor's performance.

The concept of evaluating your doctor may seem a bit formal for a patient to do, but it's a long-standing practice in medicine. In fact, several national organizations have developed physician scorecards. If you have Blue Cross insurance, for example, your plan may already have extensive empirical data on your physician; Premera Blue Cross in Washington State has a quality scorecard which measures several areas of performance, including patient satisfaction. And HealthGrades rates hospitals and nursing homes, as well as doctors. (Physician evaluations are publicly available for a fee at HealthGrades.com.)

A quick note on these scorecards: while they can be helpful, keep in mind that some are biased. For example, they may take into consideration a doctor's willingness to prescribe only from a list of preferred medications—a factor that saves the insurance company money but does nothing for you.

More important, however, these prefab report cards are missing one important ingredient: you! To overcome this omission, I have developed a model below to help you grade the doctor by your own evaluative measures. This is not a scientifically tested scorecard, and not all the categories may be equally important to you; it's just meant to help you form your own opinions about different aspects of your doctor's performance in caring for you.

In fact, I have used this system to rate my own physicians, and I can tell you that some of them have not passed the test. We've all chosen losers— even me, and even after all my experience. (When that happens, get a second opinion—something I'll discuss in a later chapter). Hopefully the scorecard I've designed and provided here will minimize the chances that you'll get stuck with a bad physician.

The process is simple. For each of the four categories listed below (doctor skills; communication; office operations; and trust and comfort), consider the individual characteristics and then rate the entire category from -1 to +2 using the following scale:

- Outstanding: +2
- Good: +1
- Average (neither good nor bad): 0
- Poor or bad: -1

Add the scores from the four categories to find your total. A doctor scoring 4 or more is probably good. But if the total score is 2 or less, consider getting a second opinion or even changing doctors. If you have given more than one *poor* ranking in any category, think carefully about whether this doctor has what it takes to keep your trust and give you quality care.

## The Doctor Scorecard

### Category 1: Physician Skills

Characteristics:

- The doctor trained at well-known hospitals or universities.
- The doctor has a good reputation with nurses and other doctors.

- The doctor is well-informed about medicine and recent medical advances.
- The doctor is well-organized.
- The doctor is confident in offering evaluations and advice.
- The doctor is concerned about maintaining health as well as curing illness.
- The doctor is comprehensive, paying attention to all your symptoms and illnesses.
- The doctor focuses on the whole patient (your life, family, and activities, as well as your illness).
- The doctor follows up on symptoms or abnormalities rather than neglecting them.
- The doctor is willing to consult with other doctors.

## Category 2: Physician and Office Communication

Characteristics:

- The doctor takes the time to listen, understands you, and does not interrupt you.
- The doctor communicates easily and speaks clearly and understandably.
- The doctor explains everything to make sure you understand.
- The doctor gives you the time you need rather than checking the clock or talking with one hand on the door.
- The doctor calls you back.
- The doctor looks you in the eye when talking to you.
- The doctor answers all your questions.
- The doctor remembers you and information about you.
- The doctor reads information you bring to the office, whether it's from the newspaper, a trade publication, or the Internet.

## Category 3: Office Operations

Characteristics:

- The doctor is on time.
- If the doctor uses a nurse practitioner or physician's assistant, the doctor actively supervises your care and will see you personally if you need or request it.

- The doctor allows you to record the visit or any advice, or lets you take notes without rushing you.
- The doctor allows you to bring family or friends to the visit so they can help participate in your care.
- The doctor provides copies of physician notes, tests, and records.
- The doctor and staff interact well with your insurance company and with other doctors' offices.

**Category 4: Your Comfort Level and the Doctor's Bedside Manner**

Characteristics:

- The doctor is caring, courteous, and respectful.
- You have confidence in the doctor.
- The doctor has a good personality, and you enjoy your office visit with him or her.
- The doctor seems dedicated and committed only to you (with no conflicts of interest).
- The doctor has compassion and sympathy for you.
- The doctor is not arrogant and can admit any mistakes or limitations in his or her knowledge.
- The doctor does not seem depressed or overworked.

Continue to observe these characteristics over time, and see if your doctor's score increases or decreases as you become more familiar with each other. If your doctor scores poorly in one or more areas, discuss this with his staff. Some problems may be easily remedied (for example, if he is often late, perhaps the staff can tell you when during the day or week he is more likely to be on time), but other issues may be impossible to correct (if he never pays attention to what you say, for instance). If there are real problems, it is best to get a second opinion or simply find another primary-care doctor.

Finally, compare your report card with one compiled by your insurance company. Understand that their report cards will be different; they measure compliance with evidence-based guidelines, which are very important to health outcomes. They'll score things like frequency of diabetic testing in patients with diabetes, or use of cardiac drugs such as ACE inhibitors, aspirin, or beta-blockers after a heart attack. They'll even score a doctor by how much money he saves them by avoiding hospital admissions or ordering fewer tests and consultations. On the other hand, your card will be more of a personal evaluation—your own estimate of the doctor's ability to make you feel comfortable and secure.

Combine these two report cards and you should have a pretty good measure of what your experience with a new doctor will be.

## Case Studies

These concepts might sound abstract, but let me tell you about a few true instances when following instincts and reacting appropriately to a physician's personal shortcomings may have saved a few lives.

**Go with Your Gut.** When a forty-year-old patient went to her primary physician with abdominal pain, the doctor just changed her diet. She went along with the plan, deferring to her doctor's quick advice, although she had a gut feeling she needed further testing. Increasingly, she suspected that something was wrong, but she waited four months before making an appointment with a stomach specialist. A colonoscopy showed colon cancer that had already spread to her lymph nodes and liver. The lesson: if your gut feeling is that you need more done, and especially if your symptoms are not getting better, get a second opinion, and get it fast! Listen to your feelings.

**Expect Respect.** A fifty-one-year-old patient developed mild back pain. When she called her doctor's office, she went through one automated question after another for five minutes, until an automated voice finally told her the office staff was too busy to take her call and instructed her to leave a message. Which she did. Three times. But after no callback in twenty-four hours, she left a different message: she was getting another doctor! If the office did not respect her enough to return her call, this was not the right physician for her. The lesson: when you do not get the respect you deserve, find another doctor who will deliver for you.

**Too Busy to Care.** Although the patient was ninety-three, he still enjoyed traveling and dancing with his wife. But his activity level was hampered when he developed an enlarged prostate. He needed surgery and contacted a urologist. The urologist scheduled the operation but never saw the patient before he went under anesthesia. After surgery, the doctor did not see him for two more days. During a follow-up office visit, the doctor did not recall he had already completed the operation until the patient reminded him—and then the doctor said, "Oh, yeah. You're right. I did it already." The patient fired the doctor the next day. The lesson: your doctor should know your treatment history, should have the results from that treatment, and should not be confused about your treatment plan.

## Advice from a Doctor-Turned-Patient

When I was in medical school at the University of Buffalo, one of my most beloved, learned, and experienced professors was Dr. Samuel Sanes, who taught me the pathology of the human body, what goes wrong in illness, and the importance of a correct diagnosis. Unfortunately, Dr. Sanes developed widespread lymphoma, a cancer of the lymph nodes, which over several years resulted in many visits with his colleagues—not as their teacher, but as their patient.

His background as an educator gave Dr. Sanes great insight into the good and the bad of his own medical care, both of which he wrote about in *Buffalo Physician*, the university's physician magazine. His articles were designed to educate former students and colleagues about how to be better doctors for their patients. When he became too weak to write, he dictated to his wife. The following recommendations, printed here by permission, are adapted from Dr. Sanes's final writings:

- **You should expect good physicians to have a friendly rapport.** Otherwise known as "bedside manner," the close relationship you have with your doctor can lead to more effective trading of information. You disclose your symptoms and concerns, and your doctor provides comprehensive information on your treatment. This healing rapport is the central tenet, indeed the trademark, of an excellent physician.
- **You should seek physicians who are reasonably on time and are personally available to you and your family.** Obviously, some tardiness can be excused if the doctor is busy with an emergency or engrossed in answering a prior patient's concerns, but if your doctor is late, he or she should at least offer an explanation. Also, you should expect to be seen by the doctor personally unless the staff warns you that he or she

is not available. Any substitute doctor, nurse practitioner, or physician's assistant should be of equally high quality.

- **Excellent physicians take all the time you need to address your concerns.** Rushed visits produce poor results.
- **You should expect doctors to introduce themselves to you and your family.** Continued interactions should be characterized by calm, concern, attentiveness, objectivity, and an intimate knowledge of your problems. Interruptions should be minimal. All questions posed by you, your family, or your friends must be listened to, evaluated, and answered.
- **The doctor must be truthful, honest, and offer complete information (no half-truths).** The doctor's thoughts and questions should be easily understood, not technical, and expressed in laymen's terms rather than medical jargon. Promises or commitments made to you or your family should be kept.
- **You should expect complete explanations of serious information or diagnoses, made by the doctor personally.** A doctor should never leave unanswered questions to nurses or staff. Doctors should use diagrams, X-rays, or printed reports to help you completely understand your illness and treatment. You must feel the doctor is willing to repeat information, if necessary, to be certain you understand what is important. Answers should be provided if you ask about unproven methods of treatment, information from the Internet, advice from friends, or newspaper articles.
- **The office should provide information about how to contact your physician at any time.** You must not feel any reluctance to call your doctor.
- **The doctor should be committed to caring for you for the entire duration of the illness and beyond, as appropriate.** You should never feel that your doctor might abandon you for any reason.
- **You should expect hope, encouragement, and support by the doctor and the staff.** A physician should never be angry with you or your family.

**Tips**

- You should know any ratings of your doctor that others have developed.
- You should use the *Surviving American Medicine* Doctor Scorecard to help you personally evaluate how well your doctor is caring for you.
- You should have high expectations for the care your doctor provides. The recommendations adapted from Dr. Sanes are excellent.

## Today's Medicine and Evaluating Your Doctor

No matter which health-care reforms are implemented by new legislation or by insurance companies, your doctor will be more stressed and subject to increased limitations on his own medical judgment as imposed by review committees, panels, and guidelines. It's very likely that many physicians will simply retire because they are unwilling to put up with the hassles of medical practice in the new health-care landscape. You may have to find new physicians, and you'll have to reevaluate how well your present or new physicians are doing in delivering quality health care. The tools I've provided in this chapter will give you a good framework for determining whether your doctors deserve your trust.

# Chapter 4

# Medical Errors and Dangerous Doctor Traits

## Medical Errors

All across the country, physicians and hospitals are busier than ever. Overhead costs have increased in practices and hospitals, resulting in fewer physicians, nurses, and staff, so doctors have been forced to care for ever-greater numbers of patients. At the same time they are expected to provide more documentation for accurate billing, oversee more administrative functions, complete more insurance requests for authorizations or review, and attend more meetings to comply with hospital or medical staff rules.

The simple fact is, in the doctor's eight-to-twelve-hour workday, she has less time than ever to spend with you. And when a doctor or nurse is rushed, that's when errors occur.

I remember on one occasion calling down to radiology to question a doctor about a report in which he had diagnosed one of my patients with an enlarged prostate. When I pressed him on it, he told me he was absolutely sure of his diagnosis.

"It's in front of the rectum, and it's huge," he told me.

"That's odd," I said. "My patient is a woman. Women don't have prostates."

As it turned out, what he had thought was a prostate gland was, in fact, a cancerous mass. He made an error because he had failed to read the request form, and that error could have been fatal for my patient.

Medical errors commonly occur, and usually they're not critical. But sometimes they can be lethal, and those are the times when you, your doctors, and your nurses must be vigilant. If you find your doctor is making errors, consider moving on.

Here are some steps that you can take to help keep your treatment error-free:

- Always bring your personal medical record with you when you go to the doctor's office or hospital so you can compare any new information you receive to your prior medical history. Definitely know your blood type to minimize the risk of receiving mismatched blood (as happened to my aunt).
- Have a complete list of the medicines you're currently taking or have taken so that your doctor can be aware of possible allergic reactions or conflicting medications. If you are told you need a new medicine, always ask, "Will this new medicine be okay with all my other medicines?" Then, to be absolutely certain, confirm with your pharmacist that the new medicine is compatible.
- Ask for the results of all your labs and X-rays to make sure they have reached your doctor's office. All too often, a test ordered by your doctor is never reported back to him, meaning serious and sometimes life-threatening abnormalities can go undetected for months. Before a doctor makes a decision about your care, ask him about all your recent results. Request a copy, read the report, and ask the doctor to explain any abnormality. (Abnormal lab results are almost always highlighted by an asterisk, bold lettering, or placement in an "out of range" column.) Then put that copy of your report in your own personal medical file (see appendix 1).
- Be cautious with physicians, nurses, or technicians who seem unaware of your history when they start your treatment. People who have not taken the time to read your record may be prone to making grave errors.

- Read up on your medications. Some physicians' offices and many pharmacies have brochures that describe in detail how medications should be taken. You can also get considerable help from the Food and Drug Administration (FDA) website, FDA.gov, and the *Physicians' Desk Reference* (available through Drugs.com/pdr or PDR.net), which details almost every drug imaginable and is frequently updated. Ask the nurse in the office to show you how to read the "contraindications" section of the medication's package insert or the printout of online information, as well as any warnings and side effects. If you are not Internet proficient, and after you understand how to look up your medicines in the *PDR*, either purchase a copy of the book in the health section of your local bookstore or have the appropriate pages copied at your doctor's office, pharmacy, or library. If you develop side effects from a medication, let your doctor's office know immediately.

- Get information about your disease from the doctor's office, the hospital, or a specialty organization such as the American Heart Association, American Lung Association, American Cancer Society, or American Diabetes Association, so that you have a basic understanding of the illness before you see your doctor. Again, the Internet is a great resource for this type of information; a good comprehensive website is WebMD.com/drugs.

- If you feel your doctor or the staff is rushing you out the door, ask them to slow down. Or ask a question to focus the doctor's attention, like, "Could you also examine my ears (or any other relevant body part) to be certain that nothing is wrong there?" or "What other diseases could this be, and what have you ruled out?"

- If you feel uneasy about something the doctor or nurse has said, speak up immediately. Ask him or her to clarify, and don't stop asking until the information has been broken down so you can follow it.

- Since four ears are better than two, always have a friend or family member with you when you talk to your doctor (or record the visit on a smart phone or small tape recorder), and get your companion's opinion afterward.

## Dangerous Doctor Traits

Everyone has a few bad traits. Some people are upstanding but always late. Others are loyal but lazy. The same is true for physicians. There are some otherwise good physicians whose few bad traits can poison a doctor-patient relationship. They key is recognizing these traits before they become a problem.

### Big Ego and Bad Attitude

A common, frustrating problem in American medicine is the physician's ego. Put simply, some doctors feel they hold a special position that excuses them from treating you respectfully. That's the root of what is often called a "God complex," and it can get in the way of your care. In dealing with her world-famous surgeon who just wasn't giving her the information she needed, one of my patients told me, "He just can't slow down to answer a question. He treated us as if we were lucky to be in his presence and shouldn't push our luck by asking annoying questions. Someday someone is going to die because of his attitude."

Arrogance isn't simply an annoyance; it's a ticking time bomb waiting to blow. The fact is, medical care is often a team effort. If your doctor won't talk to you, your doctor probably won't talk to your other doctors either. This kind of arrogance reduces the flow of information—a potentially fatal problem.

### Failing to Keep Up with New Treatments and Advances

Medicine in the twenty-first century is changing extraordinarily quickly. The way I learned to take care of patients when I was in medical school has improved dramatically, and there are new treatments discovered every day. To be a good physician, each and every doctor must stay abreast of the new approaches, the new drugs, and even the new diseases. Nothing is as it was when a doctor graduated from medical school, even if that doctor graduated just last year.

There are many ways a doctor can keep up with advances in medicine. He can read journals, attend medical conferences, work with clinical trials—even just have lunch with other doctors to discuss their work. In every medical specialty, national guidelines are rewritten every month to include new advances that must be considered in caring for each patient.

How can you tell if your doctor is slipping behind the state of medical knowledge? Ask. The following questions can help reveal how well your doctor is keeping up with the advances that might affect you:

- Can you tell me about the new advances in my disease?
- When will I be able to use these new treatments or tests?
- What national guidelines apply to my illness? Where can I go to read them?

You can also get a second opinion. Ask a consulting physician about his impression of your initial doctor. Find out if your doctor is considered cutting-edge or old-school.

Other resources include patient support groups (you can often find these at your local hospital or university medical center—like a breast cancer support group, for example) and voluntary, disease-specific health-care organizations (like the American Diabetes Association or the American Cancer Society). Both types of groups have meetings filled with patients, nurses, family members, and even other physicians who meet to discuss the most current trends. This is information you can bring with you to your own physician. If your doctor doesn't know about support groups or voluntary health-care organizations for your illness and is unwilling to do a little research on your behalf, look for someone new.

As for doctors who do their own research, that's usually a good sign. Research doctors usually (but not always) have a comprehensive knowledge of all the modern techniques. Just keep in mind that these doctors can be ultrascientific and often have a more difficult time communicating with their patients. You may need to be persistent with your questions.

**Conflicts of Interest**

Ideally you want your physicians to be making calls based solely on what they deem best for your condition, and usually that's what they do. But in rare cases, they are serving other interests as well—often economic ones! Here are some situations in which a doctor might make a call other than what's best for you. More important, here are questions you can ask to figure out if your doctor is motivated by anything other than your well-being:

- Insurance companies may have restricted lists of tests, drugs, or treatments for which they will pay. Your doctor may decide not to order a test or drug for you because your insurance company has told the doctor it won't pay for it. Ask, "Are there tests or treatments that I should have that the insurance isn't going to cover? What are they, how much do they cost, and how much better are they than what the insurance company *will* pay for?"

- Insurance companies sometimes provide performance incentives to reduce the number of tests, treatments, or medicines that doctors prescribe. In other words, the fewer expensive tests the doctor orders, the more likely the insurance company will be to continue to refer patients to the doctor and give the doctor a bonus at the end of the year. A doctor may not order a test you need in order to improve his own insurance company or IPA scorecard. Don't be afraid to ask a direct question: "Are there tests or treatments which are very expensive, but that I should have? Are you not ordering them because the insurance company or IPA doesn't want you to?" Write down the answer and date it, so the doctor knows you are keeping records. That fact may be all the doctor needs to know to push him to request the needed care.

- Insurance companies pressure doctors and hospitals to discharge patients from hospitals earlier than needed. Ask the doctor, "If I were your relative, would you send me home now or keep me a few extra days? What are the risks if you send me home now?"

- Doctors may refer you to consultants or specialists based on payback—gifts or money given as a thank-you for the referral. Find out if the specialist to whom you're being sent is one the doctor would use for his own care. Ask, "Have you ever used this doctor for yourself or a family member or friend?"

- Your doctor may prescribe a specific medicine because a pharmaceutical company is pushing the doctor to do so—offering gifts and/or giving money in exchange for prescriptions written. Ask, "Is there any reason why you are using this particular drug? Is there an incentive to prescribe it? Is it the best one for me? Is there a national guideline that says this drug is best for my condition?"

- Your doctor may select treatments or tests based on his or her financial interest in an outside company. Some doctors own shares in labs, imaging centers, or hospitals. When you pay for tests there, the doctor is taking part of the profit. Ask, "Doctor, do you own any shares in the testing, X-ray, or surgical facility that you are sending me to? Why are you referring me to that center, rather than to the hospital or a different center?"
- Some doctors admit a patient to a clinical trial solely because they have contracts requiring a certain number of enrolled patients, or because the study contributes to the doctor's academic promotion or tenure. Ask, "Do you receive a payment for enrolling me in this clinical trial? Do you have to enroll a certain number of patients in this trial? If so, why is this trial better for me than standard care?" Doctors are obligated to answer these questions honestly. Some physicians (or their research coordinators) will volunteer this information without you asking, but most won't.

Finally, remember that a second opinion can always help reassure you that your doctor's call is correct. Many HMOs and PPOs will discourage second opinions, and it's possible you might have to pay for the second opinion out of your own pocket, but consider this: a small monetary investment to pay for a second opinion might be worth the peace of mind of knowing you're getting the right care.

## Doctors Change

Many people have the same doctor for the run of that doctor's medical career. But doctors, like everyone else, can change over time. It's not uncommon for a person to walk into the office of a kind, caring physician they've known for years only to find the doctor curt, distracted, and angry.

What causes these changes? It could be a number of factors. Some doctors become ill themselves, and what you're witnessing is a side effect of their treatment. Others get injured, develop chronic pain, or begin abusing drugs or alcohol. As they reach a certain age, signs of senility or Alzheimer's disease may surface. And in some cases, the pressures and demands of hospitals, pharmaceutical companies, and insurance companies may make a doctor simply "burn out."

If you suspect something's changed with your doctor, bring it up with the nurses or with other patients. Find out whether this is a rare occurrence— we all have bad days—or whether everyone has noticed the shift. Check with the hospital where your doctor has privileges and see if they've had any complaints. But keep in mind, a lack of formal complaints by others doesn't mean your own funny feeling about the doctor is all in your head. If you feel as though something is wrong, it probably is. Get a second opinion to check it out. And that holds true across the board.

Trust your instincts. They're what keep you alive.

## Tips

- Always be on the lookout for medical errors and report them immediately to the doctor's office or hospital.
- Use the nine steps in **Medical Errors** watching for the four **Bad Traits** to reduce the likelihood of a medical error in your care.
- Check out your doctor periodically, watching for the development of bad traits, especially conflicts of interest.

## Contemporary Medicine and Medical Errors

One of the goals of health-care reform is to reduce costly and harmful medical errors. Promoting use of electronic health records by hospitals and medical offices will reduce errors in drug ordering, duplication of testing, and treatments outside national guidelines. Regulatory requirements that mandate the disclosure of physician interests in laboratories, radiology programs, and surgical centers will help reduce conflicts of interest, or at the very least make patients aware of them.

But just as there is pressure to lower the costs of health care and reduce physician income, so, too, will there be increased physician investment in profitable joint ventures and companies that may increase conflicts of interest that lead to overuse or misuse of tests or treatments.

If you have an uncomfortable feeling that your doctor isn't ordering the right treatments for you, ask the tough questions. Ask him to explain the reasoning behind his recommendations; his answer can provide hints that a second opinion or even a new primary-care physician may be needed. The state medical board may have information about whether your suspicions might be true. Government agencies are becoming more vigilant in attempting to help protect patients. Remember, with changes in medicine, physicians have less income and also less time with patients. These changes can foster physician self-promotion, medical errors, and even fraud.

# Chapter 5

# How to Use the Internet for Better Medical Care

In this chapter, I'll tell you how to use the Internet to get information about your illnesses or maintaining your health, which are the subjects you should discuss with your doctor for effective communication. The more *good* information you have, the better your health-care team (you, your physician, the medical staff, and your insurance plan) can treat you and keep you well.

There's been a revolution in medical care in the last two decades, largely as a result of genetic research, drug development, new treatment and imaging technology, and improved methods of delivering care. But another important factor has been the use of information technology in patient and physician education and in the operations of the health-care system. Throughout this book I discuss specific websites where you will find critical information to make decisions about your medical care.

## How Your Doctor Uses the Internet

Every year physicians are using the Internet more frequently—not only after office hours but throughout the day, when online information can help them make moment-to-moment decisions about patient care. If you have very dedicated doctors, they will search the National Library of Medicine database for recent publications about your disease and its treatment. Most physicians also use their national association websites or similar sources as guidelines for managing diseases. Communication with other physicians is facilitated by e-mail or messaging to referring or consulting offices, and some practices will even e-mail or message you about test results or appointments. Sometimes a doctor's office will allow patients to ask questions via e-mail or messaging, but remember that such communications do not have the privacy protections that you want in your health care. The new laws HIPAA and HITECH make it illegal for physicians to use regular e-mail to give you private health information, and they require encryption for doctor-patient communication. The messaging systems that are part of many electronic health records and many hospital information technology systems may enable you to privately and securely communicate with your doctor.

Increasingly, medical offices are investing in electronic records that can completely replace paper patient charts. Even with the sophisticated (and very expensive) electronic records my colleagues and I now use in our offices, we are still dependent some of the time on paper records and results.

## Using Your Computer as a Medical Tool

To begin with, use your computer to check out your current doctor or a doctor you are considering for primary-care or specialty consultation. (See chapter 1 for advice on how to do this.) What you find out will help you in your relationship with your doctor. Then go to your hospital and insurance company websites and check them out too.

When communicating with your doctor's office, your hospital, or even your insurance company, ask if you can use a private messaging system for logistical questions. This includes making appointments, finding out what to bring to a visit, requesting copies of medical records, and ascertaining when follow-up is needed. I recommend *receiving* your medical records by fax, mail, or pickup at the office, rather than e-mail, to be certain that privacy is optimized. And be careful what you say in any e-mail to your doctor or hospital, since the message could be misdirected, or read by nonmedical personnel.

Most important, you should use the Internet to get information beyond what your physician has provided to more completely understand your illness and medicines, disease prevention, recent advances relevant to your care, and any available clinical trials. Learning how to search the web efficiently, so you quickly find the most authoritative medical information, can give you a positive attitude about this important resource, rather than leaving you lost and overwhelmed by unimportant, irrelevant, or misleading websites.

## Who Uses the Internet?

Nearly everyone uses the Internet to get health-care information—either personally or through family. Of my patients under age sixty-five, 75 percent have a computer—but 75 percent of my patients sixty-five or over have computers too. More than 80 percent of my patients—both over and under age sixty-five—have Internet access either personally or through their family. Over half my patients have researched their medical conditions online without my having recommended a website to them. So I am confident that everyone has the ability to get information from the Internet, regardless of age or even education. In the absence of personal or family resources, your local hospital or library can provide these services for you, and you will have a new partner on your health-care team.

Therefore, even as I urge you to find reliable online information to supplement what your doctor has told you, you've probably already been doing it. More than 75 percent of my patients ask me for further guidance about where to look on the Internet. Whether or not you have already tried it, you may still benefit from knowing which medical websites are most useful and what to do with the information you find there.

The sheer number of the online information sources can make any search daunting. As I was told by my sixty-five-year-old, computer-proficient patient with prostate cancer, "I just got burned out looking for advice online." He was understandably overwhelmed by the mix of good, informative sites; "weirdo" sites advocating totally unproven methods for personal profit; blogs by frustrated patients; sites documenting research that was promising but inappropriate for his situation; and sites with very little information at all. So here's where I tell my patients to look.

## General Medical Information

In researching the Internet for information about health or disease, most people get lost in a bottomless pit of websites: some good, some bad, some poorly disguised advertisements, and most completely irrelevant. If you plug any health-care topic into a search engine, you'll find millions of sites mentioning the topic and at least twenty pages that are more relevant.

You could spend several years searching through all those sites before finding the one with the most practical, helpful information for your situation. It's better to start with five to ten excellent sites about the particular disease or aspect of health you're interested in. (Note that you should generally avoid sites that promote entirely alternative medicines, since they are really just advertisements. If you visit one, be sure to validate any recommendations with your own doctor before using any products or procedures promoted on the site.)

Here are my recommended websites for general medical information and for information about specific diseases as well. You will notice that these sites are mostly sponsored by the federal government, national nonprofit health-care organizations, or universities. Since the organizations that sponsor these sites have very strict, objective criteria for what constitutes *good* information, you can have more confidence in what you have read there and you can trust the recommendations. This is not true of the content of websites sponsored by people who have things to sell you or who are promoting a particular political viewpoint. Shop for your online information carefully, and don't get burned.

- For patient information from the National Library of Medicine: MedLinePlus.gov.
- For general and disease-specific information: WebMD.com.
- For consumer information and newsletters from Harvard University: InteliHealth.com and Health.Harvard.edu.
- For general information on medicine and certain specific diseases: MayoClinic.com.
- For American Academy of Family Practice-approved policies regarding your care (for example, vaccinations and screening): AAFP.org.
- For recent medical publications about specific diseases, consider using the National Library of Medicine: NCBI.nlm.

nih.gov. Search all databases by typing in the disease name or health topic, and try to narrow it to diagnosis, treatment, or guidelines. You'll see a long series of titles; click on a title for a short abstract of the article. The abstracts can be confusing because of the medical terminology, but you can print any abstracts you find interesting and take them in to your doctor, who can help decipher them. A medical librarian in your community hospital can help you too.

- For guidelines on treating or evaluating your illness, try the National Guidelines Clearinghouse: Guideline.gov.

## Information on Specific Diseases

If you've already been diagnosed with an illness, you still might want to start your research with the general sites above, learning what you can about your illness of interest. Then search for further information at some of the following websites:

- For heart disease or high blood pressure, go to the websites of the Food and Drug Administration (FDA.gov/hearthealth), the American Heart Association (AmericanHeart.org), or the National Heart, Lung and Blood Institute (NHLBI.nih. gov).
- For arthritis, try the Johns Hopkins arthritis website (Hopkins-Arthritis.org) or the website of the National Institute of Arthritis and Musculoskeletal and Skin Diseases (NIAMS. nih.gov).
- For stroke, go to the Washington University Medical Center in St. Louis website (StrokeCenter.org).
- For allergy or asthma, search the website of the American Lung Association (LungUSA.org) or the Centers for Disease Control, which emphasizes environmental allergies (CDC. gov/health/asthma).
- For diabetes, you can find information at the website of the American Diabetes Association (Diabetes.org).
- For mental health or depression, go to the National Institute of Mental Health website (NIMH.nih.gov) or the National Mental Health Association website (NMHA.org).

- For cancer information, go to the websites of the National Cancer Institute (Cancer.gov), the American Cancer Society (Cancer.org), the Association of Comprehensive Cancer Centers (ACCC-Cancer.org), or for guidelines for evaluation or treatment, the National Comprehensive Cancer Network (NCCN.org). For information and support, go to the websites of the Cancer Support Community (CancerSupportCommunity. org) and Cancer Care (CancerCare.org).
- For clinical trials, go to ClinicalTrials.gov.

## What to Do with Information from the Internet

After you have found information that you think will be helpful, read it twice to be sure you understand it, and then make a list of questions to ask the doctor on your next visit. Take the list to the doctor's office to be certain the information is applicable to your disease or condition. After looking at it, your physician may be able to refer you to additional resources on the web.

If you are attending support groups, discuss what you have found in your research to see if other patients might have input about what you've read that would put it into better context. They may also suggest additional sites that they have used. But remember that many websites contain poor or erroneous recommendations. Keep a log of the sites you have visited without finding anything useful, so you don't keep going back to them again.

## What Not to Do on the Internet

The Internet can give you tons of data rapidly—so much that it actually confuses rather that illuminates your understanding. Certain activities are likely to give you *bad or confusing* results:

- **Using "find a doctor" tools on the web.** This is likely to get you to doctors who have sponsored the site or paid for the referral. At a hospital website, all the doctors will usually have to be listed for referral, whether they are good or bad, young or old, experienced or brand-new, "lab rat researchers" or really good clinical doctors.

- **Reading everything in a general disease search.** If your search turns up a thousand matches for a disease or treatment, skip everything except those from very reputable sources like universities, research centers, the National Institutes of Health, or well-known treatment centers.

- **Believing everything you read on blogs.** Many blogs are supported by people with biased, nonobjective views, so any information on those sites should be considered suspect. That said, some blogs occasionally have useful information which can give you ideas from other patients about treatments or symptoms—ideas that you can discuss with your own doctor. In general, be skeptical of what you read until you have checked it out with the nurses or physician. Blogs on well-respected sites (WebMD and Medscape, for examples) can be trusted; others are often questionable.

- **Believing everything in web advertisements.** These are designed to sell you products, and frequently these products are not proven to be effective or even safe. However, you can learn a lot from the drug information pages on pharmaceutical company websites. Usually included within those websites are the results of clinical trials on the drug, its side effects, information about dosing and drug stability, and clearly written guidelines for patient use. My patients frequently are helped by use of these sites.

## Tips

- Use your computer often to search for information about your doctor, your hospital, and your illnesses or symptoms. If you get stuck trying to find information, ask your family or librarian. If you get stuck trying to understand the information you find, ask your nurse or doctor.
- Check with your physicians about any information you find to be certain it is relevant to your condition.
- Verify with your doctor any patient reports from blogs.

- Remember to focus on what you need: the right doctors, the right insurance, the right treatments, and the right disease-prevention plan.

## Contemporary Medicine and the Internet

If there is one thing that today's medicine and health-care changes are counting on, it's that you can and will use the Internet to help with your care. Why? Since doctors have less time to discuss things with individual patients and their families, and since medical office and hospital staffs are cutting back on personnel, you will have to take more responsibility for your own care. Fortunately, the Internet is at your fingertips to help you ascertain that you're getting the right treatments and to give you confidence in your health-care team. And for you and your doctors to communicate effectively, you need a system in place to help their overburdened offices get you what you need.

Each year you may have to make decisions about which health plan to use, where to get your medicines, and which doctors to choose. Use the Internet as a tool in your decision making so you can have confidence in your choices.

# Chapter 6

# Nurse Practitioners and Physicians' Assistants

The truth is that at some time or another you will receive part of your medical care from mid-level providers or physician extenders: nurse practitioners (NPs) or physicians' assistants (PAs). Already in many primary-care physicians' and specialists' offices, it is very common to use an NP or PA to handle simple problems like a sore throat, a cut, a urinary infection, or follow-up of diabetes or hypertension. The use of these mid-level providers is now common in HMOs and PPOs as well as private insurance plans. When ambulatory-care organizations (ACOs) become more widespread, NPs and PAs will be an even more integral part of the physician-patient relationship. They also will increasingly take on the role of care coordinators to maintain better patient health without having to use inpatient hospital care.

**The advantages for the physician** are that an NP or PA saves time spent with you for routine checkups or simple therapy so that the physician may spend additional time on more serious patient problems. The NP or PA can develop a very close supportive relationship with the patient, sometimes even closer than the doctor. The disadvantages for you, the patient, are that the doctor feels more distant from you, you do not develop as close a relationship with the doctor, and the medical practice feels more like a factory or "patient mill." The NP or PA might overlook problems, or make errors if the illness becomes more complex than he or she has been trained to handle. The NP or PA always requires close oversight by the physician. Your burden is to recognize when that oversight has been insufficient for your condition or care.

**The advantages for the patient** are that there is often faster access to care from an NP or a PA, especially if the physician is overscheduled or stressed by administrative responsibilities—and faster care often means less suffering. And if you are one of those patients who feels anxious or intimidated when you see a doctor, you might respond more positively to a mid-level provider. The disadvantage for you is that sometimes an NP or PA has insufficient supervision to take care of what may actually be a more serious illness. You might feel that if you are not seeing the physician, your quality of care is worse (and sometimes it really is). Errors may take place if the mid-level provider is not adequately supervised or does not adequately report back to the physician. Some patients lack confidence in a mid-level provider, which translates into a loss of confidence in the doctor and the practice. Plus the turnover rate for mid-level providers is usually greater than that of physicians, so continuity of care may be lost as well.

Do NPs and PAs have good clinical judgment, just like physicians? Generally, yes. Both types of mid-level providers receive considerable training and must pass certification examinations to obtain their license. In most circumstances, they have excellent clinical judgment, but in some cases they do not. Doesn't this sound very similar to physicians?

It may be hard to determine whether you can totally trust the NP or PA in your physician's office. Since the turnover rate at that position is higher, just when you do develop some confidence in your doctor's NP or PA, he or she may leave the practice. Other patients may have had favorable or bad experiences with the mid-level providers in an office you are using, so don't be afraid to ask around while you are waiting for an appointment.

One of my friends, Karen, had been with her internist for fifteen years. Just after informing Karen that she had diabetes and needed insulin, her doctor told her he was hiring a nurse practitioner and would only be available to Karen if she had a severe problem. As she complained to me, "Here I am, sixty-one years old, just dumped by my doc." But after she looked at the NP's credentials, Karen was satisfied that her care would still be good, so she stayed with the doctor … until one day, when she realized that the doctor had not seen her in eighteen months. Karen requested an appointment with her internist to find out how she was handling the diabetes and what would be in store for her in the long run—and that's when she was told she could not get an appointment to talk to him. Karen's doctor had failed an important test: being available to a patient when only his advice could confidently answer his patient's concern. So Karen left that doctor—a good decision for her, and one that can be an example for you about when to trust your doctor and nurse practitioner.

NPs or PAs have not received the same intense training or the same exposure to medical errors and problems in medical judgment as the physician. Therefore, you must be cautious and observant when your only care comes from a mid-level provider—especially if your disease is serious, your symptoms are severe, or your symptoms are persistent following initial therapy. In such circumstances you need to be certain there is very close supervision of your care and constant interaction between your doctor and the NP or PA. And it's critical that you can actually talk to your physician when you feel a need to do so.

## The Bottom Line

If you truly like the doctor, and the doctor uses an NP or PA, give the doctor and assistant a chance to prove that they can be responsive to your requests and respectful of your need to see the doctor personally when desired. If you can't get in to see your doctor when you need to, or if you are frustrated by your interactions with the NP or PA, consider getting a second opinion or changing to another practice altogether.

## Tips

- Check the training and experience of the physician's NP or PA by requesting his or her curriculum vitae (or resume or biography) from the office staff, the nurse, or even the doctor. You should review the credentials and CV of a mid-level provider just as you would that of a doctor (see chapter 1).
- Ask the secretary about the certification, continuing education credits, and licensure of the mid-level provider.

- Ask the staff or nurses about office policies and procedures regarding which patients see the NA or PA versus the physician. Ask how often the doctor interacts with the NP or PA.
- Ask if you can see the physician personally whenever you feel it is necessary, or whenever you don't feel confident about the care or advice provided by the mid-level provider.
- Talk to your fellow patients about their experiences with the mid-level provider and with the doctor as well. Do those patients feel confident, well cared for, and comfortable in those relationships? How often have they seen the physician rather than the NP or PA? Do they really know the doctor at all? When they asked to speak to the doctor about a problem, how responsive were the staff and the doctor?
- If you are dissatisfied with the NP or PA, ask for a personal visit with the doctor to discuss the problem. If no solution is offered, get a second opinion or find a new doctor. Advise your health plan representative of your dissatisfaction and the reasons for changing practices; they may suggest other physicians for you to consider. You must have confidence in all your doctors *and* their mid-level providers, if they use them.
- Use the *Surviving American Medicine* Doctor Scorecard for the nurse practitioner or physician's assistant, just as you did for the doctor.

If you notice any of these clues, consider discussing your dissatisfaction with the office or getting a second opinion:

- You never see the doctor.
- The doctor is not in the office when you are seeing the NP or PA.
- You are not getting better.
- The NP or PA has not discussed disease prevention with you.
- The NP or PA is unaware of the national guidelines for treating your condition.
- When the doctor sees you, he or she seems unfamiliar with your case.
- The doctor seems distant or burdened by having to see you.

## Today's Medicine and Mid-Level Providers

Not only will efficient health care benefit from increased use of NPs or PAs, there is no way we can meet Americans' health-care needs without them. The question is not whether your doctor will use an NP or PA, but how many of them your doctor will be supervising. One? Two? Five? Ten? And at what point will your physician be so overworked that you don't get the supervision you need? With changes in contemporary medicine, it's becoming your responsibility to recognize when you're not getting enough physician (as opposed to NP or PA) attention.

# Chapter 7

# Communicating with Your Doctor

Unfortunately, the opportunities for you to talk with your doctor are diminishing. In this chapter, I will suggest ways to improve communication so that when you get that opportunity, it is more efficient and comprehensive and results in better care.

In the past, physicians had plenty of time to talk to you. They saw fewer patients overall, the pace was slower, and the technology simpler. What the physician had to tell you and what needed to be written down took much less time. There was even time for casual conversation, a hug or a pat on the back, and learning a bit more about the doctor and the nurse.

However, with today's health-care changes and managed-care plans, physicians have to do far more tedious work: filling out forms, completing electronic medical records, and administering an increasingly regulated business—the office. And this is in addition to the time they spend face-to-face with you. But even if you understand why your doctor is stressed and rushed, you probably need more of her time and attention to completely understand your condition, tests, and treatments and to get preventive medicine.

Why is it important to learn to ask all your questions, get all your problems addressed by your doctor, and understand everything she has told you? Because a serious disease or condition could be smoldering behind any mild symptom or little problem. Taking care of an illness when it's in its earliest stage is easier and can leave you with fewer side effects or disabilities than if you wait until the condition is more advanced. But if you can't communicate effectively, you could miss out on curing a potentially dangerous problem.

You might be thinking, *I've been going to doctors' offices for years. Why should I consider changing how I've been talking to doctors? I'm still fine.* Well, even if you've gone to the doctor a hundred times, if you've gotten poor attention while overlooking important decisions or preventive treatments, you've been getting inadequate care. The fact that the care is consistent doesn't make it any better unless you adopt some new approaches, skills, or aids to treatment. So consider changing how you interact with your doctor to improve the overall quality of your health care.

## Asking Questions

When asked a question, doctors nearly always listen and answer. This is an important tip! If you bring a list of questions with you, and you ask those questions quickly and efficiently, your doctor usually will take the time to answer every one. Doctors almost always try to make enough time for you if they know you need it. For example, my staff knows that certain people always come with long lists of questions, and they schedule an extra five to ten minutes for those patients' appointments.

Furthermore, when my patients arrive with a list of questions, I'm much more diligent about working down the list and making certain that I've answered all of them. Many times, I'll even write the answers down for my patients on their own sheet of paper. This has been a godsend for the ones who were nervous and could not remember what they wanted to ask. Have you ever been so nervous at one of your doctor appointments that you have forgotten something? If so, always make a list of every question you want to ask, and do not hesitate to ask every question you have.

When I visit my own doctor, I always forget some questions if I have not written them down (and I am surely less anxious than the typical patient). Sometimes I'll think of a question to ask my physician several weeks before an appointment, and yet I cannot remember it when I get to the office. I'm certain most of my patients have similar experiences, because often upon

This allows—and often requires—you to be direct with your physician. If he refuses to implement your choice of treatment, he must explain his reasons fully. (For example, a doctor will usually refuse to continue opiate drugs or medicines for anxiety if a patient does not have symptoms that warrant their use.) If your opinion is not being respected, if your wishes are not being followed, you should seek a second opinion to get the full scoop: complete information, the proper tests, and a full choice of treatments.

Almost every health plan stresses the importance of the patient making the final decision about his or her own medical care. And I know of no health plan that refuses a second opinion to you if you request one (although some plans restrict your choice of doctors for the second opinion).

How can you be direct without offending your doctor? A good physician does not consider a direct request to be confrontational. Before you get to the office, write down the language you want to use to impart the tone you wish to convey: decisive, helpful, collaborative, supportive, state-of-the-art, comprehensive, cautious, and hopeful.

An often-overlooked aspect of the doctor-patient relationship involves mutual respect. If you are more respectful of your physician, she will react in kind. With a mutually respectful relationship, you can expect more from her with less objection or haste. If you want to establish a better relationship with your doctor and avoid the appearance of being offensive or too direct, here are some helpful hints: dress nicely; make sure you are well-groomed and clean; act politely and with dignity; and be prompt (or let the office know if you will be late). Your attitude should always be reflected back in your doctor's attitude. If it is not, mention it to the doctor's staff.

When you talk to the doctor, nothing important should be omitted. A good physician will be interested not only in your health, injury, illness, or chronic conditions, but also in disease prevention, your activities, and your personal future aspirations. Communication keeps the doctor-patient team focused not only on treatment, but also on fulfillment in life.

## Patient Portals

With the increasing availability of electronic health records, some institutions and physician offices are now using patient portals—an electronic method of communication between a patient and an office, hospital, or clinic. A portal can include only digital messages (a message basket), or it can also provide access to the patient's electronic record so he or she can see actual laboratory or X-ray results and even physician's notes.

Why not just e-mail the doctor's office? The reasons involve security and legality (the Health Insurance Portability and Accountability Act of 1996 – HIPAA). Since e-mail is not secure (it is not encrypted or firewall protected), it is more prone to hacking or even just inadvertent sending (or forwarding) to the wrong recipient. E-mails about your health concerns can include private information you do not want other people to see. Logically, therefore, medical information should be conveyed through a secure system with privacy safeguards.

That's why Congress passed laws requiring doctors and hospitals to use only secure systems, and prohibiting their use of simple e-mail for communication. Those laws, known as HIPAA and HITECH, restrict how health-care providers can digitally talk with you. In contrast to e-mail, which is easy to hack into and often inadvertently compromised (resulting in private health information leaks and even identity theft), messaging systems are encrypted, password protected, and firewall secure. Systems that meet the federal regulations are called HIPAA- and HITECH-compliant, and they give you the peace of mind that your communications will not be read by people wanting to steal your identity or your private health information. These messaging systems (often provided as part of electronic health records) are as simple to use as e-mail, so you shouldn't be fearful of the process.

As physician practices become busier and we all become more "tech-savvy," having a communication portal at your physician's office can be a real convenience. A patient facing a serious illness can have more peace of mind knowing he or she can send a message to the doctor 24/7. Just think—when you read about a new advance and wonder if it might apply to you, you can send your doctor a message any time of the day or night, so you don't risk forgetting about it at your next visit. Or when you need to change an appointment or get a medicine refill, you won't have to wait on hold with the office or try to get through to the right person to make your request; you can just send a quick message and get a reply later that day or the next. You can find out whether your blood test was okay, or even get a copy of the result, without spending an hour reaching a nurse by phone only to hear, "I'll have to call you back about that test when I find it."

Since communication portals can help in making your medical care more efficient, you might want to consider the availability of such a system when you're looking for a new doctor or specialist. If you like your physician but she doesn't have a portal system, ask the office manager if the doctor would consider putting such a portal in place—and ask other patients in the waiting room to make that request too, if they agree it would be helpful.

### Tips

- Bring lists of all your current health problems and questions.
- Bring your personal medical record to your first doctor visit.
- Before you come to the office, fill out all available forms and your review of systems.
- Be prepared to take notes or record your office visit.
- Always consider bringing a friend or a family member to the doctor's office.
- Ask for a copy of the results of any laboratory tests or X-rays and a copy of the visit note.

## Communication in Contemporary Medicine

A fundamental tenet of health-care reform is that better communication with patients empowers them to get better quality medicine. Today, physicians and hospitals are experiencing two revolutions that affect you and your care.

First, medical providers are under pressure to use electronic health records in order to improve quality, and to be monitored to measure their quality. That is one reason to choose doctors and hospitals with electronic record systems (besides the fact that when you get an electronic copy of your records, you can actually read it). These systems can give you information that leads to better advice to you and better questions for you to ask your nurses and doctors during follow-up visits. These systems also can include a patient portal so you can send important messages to your nurses or doctors.

Second, medical providers are being asked to provide more comprehensive care to more patients in less time than ever before. Remember when doctors used to take the time to get to know you and your family? Now they are rushed out of the examining room to answer calls from the hospital, stressed patients, or nurses with questions. And that's assuming you can even get a timely appointment to begin with.

So it's imperative that you find a way to get the most out of your brief doctor visit. And you should find a way to communicate with your medical offices more efficiently so you get rapid, understandable, comprehensive medical advice. By having a good list of questions, another set of ears to hear the answers and advice, and electronic aids to convey your questions and concerns, you can improve the quality of your care and your satisfaction with it.

# Chapter 8

# Keeping Your Medical Information Private

For my patient George, who was eighty years old and facing prostate cancer therapy, his biggest concern was not his illness but his privacy. "My sister is seventy-three, and she's always been after my money," he explained. "Now she'll find out about this, and she's just going to start a vigil, waiting for me to die. She can't wait to get my house."

I promised George that my office would not give any information to his sister, and that my entire staff would know she was off-limits. George lived another six happy years, his quality of life unspoiled by disagreements with his sister, who didn't learn of George's condition until one month before his death. Keeping a promise to our patient was a bond between all our staff and George.

A basic principle of medical ethics is that any patient's health care is totally private and confidential. This principle is legally regulated on the state and federal levels so that everything in your medical record is private; it cannot be sent to anyone without your consent. This chapter will help you understand these privacy regulations and how to keep all your information confidential.

Why is everyone regulating medical privacy so strictly? It is because your health-care information has become very valuable to businesses and marketing agencies. Many companies, including drug distributors and pharmaceutical manufacturers, are anxious to get this information; it helps them understand how to advertise more effectively, how to develop new products, and how to make higher profits. And they can sell important information about you and your medical care to other businesses. Potential employers want your information too, since they are more reluctant to hire you if you have health problems.

If you want to protect your privacy, never allow your information to be used in any type of marketing or business promotion. Occasionally, a hospital may ask to use your information for charitable campaigns or for development of a new program at the institution. For example, your information might be used to develop a list of patients with your disease who might contribute to research or prevention programs, or to develop a new treatment center at the hospital. Some patient lists are developed so the hospital can send the patients educational materials or updates on advances in treatment of their disease. However, that information can also be used to advertise new drugs to those patients. The bottom line is, you should be very suspicious and cautious—not only about identity theft, but also about medical history theft.

When you last entered a hospital or began treatment in an office, how many forms did you have to fill out? Did it take five minutes? Ten? Thirty? Did you read all the fine print? Many of these forms allow the physician or hospital to send your information to other health-care providers and offices, while others permit the physician or hospital to obtain information from your previous medical visits. Still others describe all the privacy rules of the office or medical center.

Every year, new federal and state regulations increase the protection of confidential information. In 2002, federal regulations were written to implement the Health Insurance Portability and Accountability Act (HIPAA) passed in 1996 and signed by President Bill Clinton, making it even more difficult for your private health information to be sent electronically or used in any way without your consent. These restrictions were again expanded in 2009 as part of the American Recovery and Reinvestment Act signed by President Barack Obama—a part now known as the Health Information Technology for Economic and Clinical Health Act (HITECH). As time passes, rule changes continue to demand closer control, better scrutiny, and increased documentation in order for a medical office or hospital to share your information with anyone.

To the extent that it prevents your information from going to the wrong people, all this regulation is good. However, a bad effect of the privacy rule is a long delay in sending your information to anyone until you give yet another signature. An even worse unintended outcome is that some health care decisions now might be made without any of the patient's prior records.

For example, suppose you are seeing a specialist for a second opinion or a consultation. That new doctor needs all your medical information from your prior doctors in order to understand your current illness and make the best recommendations for your treatment. Will any information be missing because one doctor's office was reluctant to send your information without a signed consent form? Is a clerk in the specialist's office reluctant to send out your records without checking with the specialist or getting another signature from you? Or will he or she just send a few things and wait for additional requests? Such delays have become more common with the tightening of privacy rules.

You can prevent a delay from possibly harming you. To expedite a consultation or a second opinion, be certain you have signed consent forms at both your prior and your new doctors' offices, and if possible, bring copies of your records to your appointment. You can get these copies from your physician or hospital by signing a request, and then you can take the information yourself to the new office. To make the process even more efficient, drop off the copies at the new office ahead of time so that the staff can organize it for the physician before your visit.

### Tips

- Ask your doctor's office or hospital if any of your medical information might be used for marketing or business activities. Then ask how you can make sure your private health information is not used for purposes other than your own necessary health care.
- Keep a copy of your medical records, as privacy regulations may prevent another office or hospital from getting them rapidly.
- When going for a second opinion, consultation, or hospital admission, phone the office to ask if you can sign consent

forms for old records in advance, so that they will be there at the time of your visit.

- When asked to fill out forms, be certain you give consent for obtaining old records and sending your records to consultants.

- Before a new doctor visit, call to make sure all your prior records have arrived for the doctor to review. By ensuring that all your records and results are present, you could save money by avoiding a repeat office visit and even unnecessary duplicate testing.

## Today's Medical Care and Privacy

Health care is becoming less efficient as physicians encounter more regulatory bottlenecks in accessing their patients' past histories and test results. Often I cannot get test results for one of my own patients if another physician ordered the test. My staff must have the patient sign more releases so that I can get to the data and make decisions.

Every patient is frustrated at having to sign so many forms again and again. But the system is demanding compliance in order to protect you against privacy breaches, even unintended ones. I expect the situation to worsen until future reforms reduce the inefficiency surrounding these regulations.

# Chapter 9

## Preventing Illness

Michael Landon was fifty-four, at the top of his career, and excited about launching his new TV series. He also had been experiencing severe abdominal pain for about a month, so he visited his primary physician. He was told he had too much stomach acid, given some antacid medications, and sent home.

But on a ski trip with his family, the pain became unbearable. He flew home early and then had blood tests and CT scans. That night he was given a grim diagnosis: pancreatic cancer that had spread to his liver. After a biopsy confirming the pancreatic adenocarcinoma, Michael underwent two standard chemotherapy treatments and decided chemo was not for him. He also attempted alternative treatments, but the tumor progressed further. He felt he was failing.

Seeking another approach, Michael had a second opinion at my center. He agreed to enter a clinical trial of an investigational new drug, liposomal chemotherapy (an anticancer drug packaged in microscopic fat bubbles).

On the way to yet another CT scan, he looked up at me, frustrated. "I was supposed to be on vacation in Mexico with my wife and kids, having fun," he said, "and here I am, waiting for another CT scan to see if my life is over. My business is great, I've got plenty of money, my family is happy, and I want to see our children grow up. I've got everything to live for, and here I am, sitting with you."

But Michael had not known about his family's dark history of colon and stomach cancers—diseases that had struck more than half his relatives. As a result, he had not been able to share that history with his doctors, who might have saved his life by performing screening tests to see if he was developing any abdominal tumors or masses, including colonoscopies (looking inside the colon), gastroscopies (looking inside the stomach and small intestine), CT scans, and tests for blood in his stool. With conventional approaches to preventing cancer, his doctors could have improved Michael's diet, given him aspirin and calcium, and advised him about avoiding high-risk lifestyle habits. If Michael had received the appropriate prevention and screening, the pancreatic cancer likely would have been found at a more treatable or curable stage, and Michael may have had the opportunity to see his children grow up. As he said to me after his remission on the new chemotherapy had come to an end, "Doc, you've got to do something to help prevent this awful disease and save others from this suffering!" (I've shared this story with the permission and encouragement of Michael's wife, Cindy.)

Every patient suffering from a serious incurable illness expresses frustration—*Why couldn't my doctor have prevented this?* It often surprises people to know that with modern medical techniques, we can, in fact, prevent or delay most diseases. Your challenge is to understand that prevention starts when you take action, and that action must continue consistently. You have to take ultimate responsibility; your doctor may be too busy to initiate your preventive care.

The very best medical treatment is the successful prevention of illness. And the next-best treatment is screening for illnesses when you are healthy, to detect any disease at its earliest stage so it can be treated and possibly cured before it progresses.

Pediatricians have spent most of the last century giving effective vaccinations to prevent childhood diseases. But only in the last ten years has American adult medicine been effective in preventing illness and screening for early stages of disease, and many insurance companies still do not pay for proven prevention and screening methods. And although medical students learn about preventing illness, most of the hands-on teaching they receive during internship, residency, and fellowship focuses on treating illnesses once they have occurred, rather than prevention and early detection.

But today, the emphasis is gradually changing. For example, although oncologists for years were totally focused on early detection and treatment of cancer, in the 1990s the National Cancer Institute supported research to determine if the drug tamoxifen could prevent breast cancer in healthy women who were at high risk of developing the disease. Women who agreed to participate in the clinical trial took either a placebo (sugar pill) or tamoxifen daily for five years. More than fourteen thousand women participated in this study, which clearly showed that tamoxifen reduced the breast cancer rate by 40 percent. For the first time, physicians who had treated patients only after cancer was diagnosed were treating healthy women to prevent cancer. This study spurred similar clinical trials focused on preventing prostate cancer, lung cancer, head and neck cancer, and colon cancer.

Why was this a paradigm shift? This new focus on prevention changed the way oncologists approached their patients. Not only did they take care of their patients with breast cancer, but also they began to discuss cancer prevention in the patients' daughters, sisters, mothers, and other female relatives, and cancer screening for all female family members. Yet still today, most gynecologists, family practice doctors, and internists are not treating women at high risk of breast cancer with tamoxifen (or raloxifene or aromatase inhibitors, which have also been shown to reduce the rate of breast cancer). While the shift in research identified ways to prevent most cancers (including prostate, colon, lung, head and neck, and rectal cancers), tragically, most doctors are not using these methods to help their patients stay healthy.

So how do you find out whether you're at risk of developing certain severe illnesses? How do you know if you should be on preventive medication or changing your habits and lifestyles to reduce your chances of getting sick?

American medicine has developed some excellent screening tests for disease. Most of us are willing to have our blood pressure, glucose level, and cholesterol measured, and women have long accepted the necessity of regular Pap smears and mammograms. More recently, CT scan screening of smokers has resulted in reduced lung cancer death rates, although doctors have been slow to implement routine screening of smokers.

Some screening tests for disease remain controversial, including CT scans to screen for coronary calcifications and cardiac disease, and total body scans (or ultrasound testing) to detect early abdominal disease (these are costly and have not been proven to reduce mortality, so discuss them with your doctor). Although men have generally accepted screening for prostate cancer by rectal examinations and, selectively, PSA (prostate specific antigen) testing, the value of regular PSA screening is under debate, since it detects many cancers that do not have to be treated immediately. (Treatment can have side effects like urine incontinence and erectile dysfunction, so be certain you discuss this with your physician.)

In seeking the best medical care from your doctors, remember this priceless rule: *the highest quality medical care includes—in this order—preventing, delaying, and screening for serious conditions.* So ask yourself these questions:

- Has your doctor discussed with you how to prevent common serious illnesses?
- Has your physician talked about preventing cancer and heart, lung, and liver disease and determined your personal risk of developing these diseases?
- Has your doctor made you aware of all the vaccinations, vitamins, nutrients, dietary changes, lifestyle improvements, and treatments that can preserve your health?
- Has your doctor discussed any of your bad habits and helped you try to stop them?
- Has your doctor told you what exercise program is best for you?[2]
- Has your doctor reviewed your family history to determine which illnesses you are likeliest to develop?
- Has your doctor given you a schedule for monitoring your preventive strategies and early detection tests to keep you healthy? (After all, that's in large part what "health" care means.)

If you cannot answer yes to all these questions, you have some work to do to stay healthy. Your challenge is to insist that your doctor help you

---

2   Exercising fifteen minutes a day reduces mortality by 14 percent and increases lifespan by three years, and every additional fifteen minutes per day reduces mortality by another 4 percent (*The Lancet*, Oct. 2011).

get all known prevention and detection tests and treatments. In addition, you want information to give to your family about their risks, prevention strategies, and where to get their own program for health.

A program for health: that is what you need in modern medicine! You have prevention strategies for your car (oil changes, inspections, preventive maintenance) and your house (termite inspections, changing air filters, and fixing plumbing or electrical problems as soon as they're discovered). You need to pay the same regular attention to your body. And you have a partner in your doctor, but she needs to be reminded to pay attention to you. That's your responsibility.

### Tips

- Add this request to the list of questions you'll take to your physician: "I want to talk about preventing disease and detecting illness early with screening tests. I want you to look at my family history and tell me what diseases I'm likely to get and how I can prevent them." After discussing your family history (a sample form you can fill out and give to your doctor is included among this book's appendixes), ask your doctor what illnesses run in your family and how to prevent them or detect them early, before they become serious.
- Ask for comprehensive lists of the tests you need to have and the lifestyle changes (diet, vitamins, exercise, bad habits, etc.) that are important for you.
- If your physician does not have good answers for you, ask her to refer you to another physician who can give you the appropriate information. This might require several specialists who can speak to your individual risks. For example, if you have a family history of cancer, your physician may refer you to an oncologist. If you have high cholesterol and a high risk of heart disease, your physician may refer you to a cardiologist. If you have a family history of blood clotting or bruising, your physician may refer you to a hematologist.

## Today's Medicine and Emphasis on Prevention

Most health plans and Medicare cover many prevention and early detection programs. Under the provisions of the Patient Protection and Affordable Care Act, private health plans are required to cover many prevention and screening services. New regulations for this act, and any further amendments (or even repeal) may change coverage, so it is important to check whether your insurance will pay for all the preventive and screening services your doctor will recommend.

Although your health insurance probably will pay your bills for these services, health plans do not require your doctors to perform them—only you can do that. As more patients are covered by insurance, however, your doctor's office is getting busier. So you have to be persistent in asking whether you have received all the prevention and screening that you need to remain healthy.

Doctor report cards—the ones developed by some insurance plans— measure how frequently doctors use some prevention/early detection methods, like Pap smears, mammograms, blood pressure control, and flu vaccinations. However, your insurance plan may not give you access to its report card, and it may not evaluate doctors' use of many risk assessments for some cancers (like lung or skin cancer), heart disease, liver disease, etc. For your purposes, though, your report card for your doctor is better than your insurance company's report card (and I have created one that you can use in chapter 2). So be certain to ask your doctor all the right questions about prevention so he'll get on the ball and do everything that's right for you.

# Chapter 10

## Predicting the Future
### Genetic Testing and Disease Risk Assessment

Jane didn't have cancer or any disease, but she was certain she was going to get cancer, because her mother had breast cancer at age thirty-five and then another cancer at age fifty, and Jane's sister had ovarian cancer at age forty. "Why do you think cancer runs in my family?" she asked me. "What can I do?"

After I counseled her about the advantages and possible risks of gene testing, Jane said she wanted to be tested. After she had blood drawn for testing mutations in BRCA1 and BRCA2, it was found that she had a mutation in BRCA2, inherited from her mother. Since Jane wanted no more children, she had her ovaries and tubes removed to prevent ovarian cancer. As sometimes happens, it was discovered that Jane's left ovary already contained a previously unsuspected early cancer, which was not detectable by exam or ultrasound since it was only 3 mm in diameter.

Jane then began tamoxifen to prevent breast cancer. In order to detect any breast cancer at its earliest stage, I started her on a program of breast exams every three months, breast mammograms and ultrasounds annually, and an MRI of the breasts every year. Jane remains happy, healthy, cancer-free, and more confident about her future. And now her children and siblings also have been tested for the mutation, with preventive strategies implemented when mutations were found.

Stories about genes and diseases are constantly in the news. Now that the human genome project, molecular biology, and our knowledge of DNA have revolutionized science, they are beginning to improve our day-to-day medical care. Not only is DNA the backbone of our genes and chromosomes and the nucleus of all our cells, but it also is the key to better treatments for disease. Most important, genes tell us what diseases you may develop.

For example, tests for BRCA1 and BRCA2 mutations (frequently detected in patients with a family history of breast or ovarian cancer, and in Jewish or Latino families) can now be analyzed to determine if you are very likely to develop breast or ovarian cancer. Other blood studies can measure your risk of other genetically inherited diseases. For example, to determine a familial tendency to develop blood clots in your legs (deep venous thrombosis) or in your lungs (pulmonary emboli), or premature heart attacks, you can have your blood tested for abnormally high cholesterol or LDL fat concentrations, high levels of the amino acid homocysteine, or mutations in clotting factor V or prothrombin. These abnormalities increase the risk of blood clots and/or heart disease. Simple medicines (such as statins, anticoagulants, folic acid, vitamin B12, and/or vitamin B6) can reduce the risk of heart attacks, strokes, and blood clots in patients with these genetic changes.

How do you determine if your case merits risk assessment or genetic testing? Ask your doctor which diseases are likely to be inherited in your family. If your physician is unfamiliar with the causes of some of those diseases, ask him to refer you to the appropriate specialist.

Genetic counselors have been trained to evaluate families in which several relatives have had identical or even similar (genetically linked or associated) diseases. If you are suspected of having a disease risk based on family history, your doctor can refer you to a genetics counselor who can discuss that risk with you and tell you whether a genetic test is available for the diseases that are common in your family. Genetics counselors also can work with your physician to give you advice for preventive medications, lifestyle changes, or screening tests to detect illness earlier, when it is more easily cured or treated.

If you need or want to be checked for gene mutations, the biggest problem you'll run into is the cost, which may be very high—up to $4,000—and may not be covered by your health insurance. There are solutions, however. First, have your doctor request authorization for the genetic test, since most insurance plans will cover it in certain circumstances. If the request is denied, have your doctor appeal the denial with the support of a specialist's recommendation. Also, ask your doctor if those tests are being evaluated for research; if so, you might be able to obtain the testing by participating in a study. (You may need the advice of a geneticist physician specialist or genetic counselor to get this answer.) If referred to such a study, make sure you will be promptly told the results of the testing and can advise your family about any abnormalities.

If there is no such study available, consider paying for the testing yourself. Your investment in genetic counseling or testing can save your life and the lives of your children by preventing premature death. As a cancer survivor once told me, "Pay for the tests instead of several dinners at restaurants. After all, it's your life, for heaven's sake." As for children, the right time for testing them for gene mutations is over age eighteen, when they are old enough to understand the ramifications and implement any necessary lifestyle changes.

A second problem you may run into with genetic testing is "insurance discrimination." If your insurance company learns that you've been found to have a gene mutation—and remember, they will be contacted to pay the bill unless you pay for it yourself—they might say you have a preexisting condition and refuse to pay for any cancer or disease that subsequently occurs.

A possible third problem is job discrimination. A prospective employer might find out that you have a gene abnormality that could raise your risk of a disease, which might then increase the employer's medical insurance premiums. (Employers are not supposed to be able to find out this information, but sometimes people disclose it unwittingly.) As a result, the prospective employer might deny you a job.

Although there are laws protecting against both insurance and employment discrimination, they have not been tested sufficiently in the courts to determine their breadth of protection. A solution to this problem is to check with your physician or genetics counselor to determine if the testing you seek is protected under state or federal law; if so, advise your doctor or counselor that you wish any genetic testing results to be kept in a separate, confidential file to prevent accidental illegal discovery by those who might request your routine medical information.

There's another possible risk involved with gene testing: if you are tested but do not have a gene abnormality, while your brother or sister is tested and found to have inherited a genetic mutation, you could feel guilty. Experiencing guilt because of failing to inherit a familial genetic mutation rarely occurs, however, and most individuals want to know if they have an increased risk so that they can take control of the problem and reduce the likelihood that they will have an illness. A genetic counselor can discuss possible emotional responses with you before you undergo testing. Most insurance plans will authorize genetic counseling, but some heavily managed health plans (like HMOs) may deny payment.

## Tips

- Ask your doctor to carefully review your family history and all your tests to evaluate whether you have a high risk of any type of disease. Ask your physician to provide you with a comprehensive plan to prevent, delay, or detect those diseases, or to refer you to a specialist who can give you a "life plan."
- Ask what types of genetic screening can determine if you have a hereditary condition causing increased risk of disease, or whether the doctor knows a genetics counselor who can tell you if such testing is possible. If your physician cannot answer this question, ask to speak to a specialist (as Jane did), or call the appropriate department at a university hospital where research into those diseases is being conducted.
- Discuss confidentiality and discrimination issues before you undergo any testing.
- If your doctor or consultant still does not provide you with clear and understandable answers, consider a second opinion. Your life and the lives of your children could depend on good physician advice.

## Contemporary Medicine and Genetic Testing

Although a cornerstone of modern medicine is disease prevention, insurance companies are slow to authorize every new genetic test. To access such tests, you must know which ones are available and which ones might help you. Use all the information-gathering tools I describe in the chapter on Internet resources to help you understand what you need.

For example, if colon cancer is present in your family, ask your doctor about all your preventive options: gene tests (HNPCC gene testing); lifestyle strategies (dietary changes to high fiber, more vegetables and fruits, and less red meat, with aspirin or Celebrex and possibly calcium); or early detection programs (periodic colonoscopy and fecal occult blood testing). Check out any online information sources, and make sure to use the resources of a disease-specific organization (like the American Cancer Society) for advice and information. Since a university or tertiary-care hospital may have a program covering the illness you're concerned about, call that facility and inquire about support programs or navigators that can help you.

With changes in health care, national guidelines for genetic testing will be more prevalent and comprehensive. Each insurance company will use some national guideline to authorize (or deny) any given test, and even small differences between different guidelines may change your access to a specific test. Use consultants, genetic counselors, and Internet information to help you understand these differences.

# Chapter 11

# Getting the Right Answers: Key Questions for Your Doctor

It's perfectly normal to be anxious about asking questions in the doctor's office—but it's not necessary. To make you more confident and to ensure that you ask the important questions and get thorough answers to them, I've listed actual questions to ask your doctor at your next office visit. These will give you the exact language you need so your doctor will pay attention to your concerns. The questions in bold type are likely to be the most important ones for many patients. My suggestion is that you write down each question that could be important to you at your next appointment. Grab some paper, your smart phone, or a tablet, and write down the precise words you want to use. That way you won't be nervous about saying them correctly, and you'll get the best answers and most complete advice. When you get into the examining room, take out your list of questions and ask them one by one. Many of my patients do this, and they get better care as a result.

Seeing a doctor can be very scary. So if you are at all apprehensive about visiting the physician (either your established one or a new one), the questions below just might be the most valuable part of this book. Review these questions to see if you have asked any of them in the past, or if they might have been overlooked. Even if you've asked and simply forgotten the information, don't be embarrassed to ask an important question again. I do it all the time with my own personal doctors.

And don't forget how advantageous it can be to have someone with you to listen to (and even write down) the answers. It helps you get the most from your office visit.

## If You Have No Illnesses or Conditions: Questions on General Health

### Staying Healthy

**What should my weight be?** What diet should I follow? Am I eating well now, or should I change my diet? What are my blood pressure, cholesterol, and fasting glucose levels?

**How much exercise do I need?** What kind of exercise? Am I fit now?

**What routine tests do I need to screen for serious illnesses?** Will they screen for cancers, heart disease, lung disease, high blood pressure, diabetes, high cholesterol, liver disease, kidney disease, bladder disease, osteoporosis, infections, oral cancer, and any other illnesses that are more common in my family? How often should I have these tests? Will your office automatically schedule them for me, or must I remind your staff that the tests are due?

**How do I prevent the most common serious illnesses—heart disease, cancer, stroke, diabetes?**

**In an emergency, whom do I call?** To which hospital will I be taken if I call an ambulance or paramedics? Will I get faster care in an emergency if I come in with paramedics or by ambulance, if I drive myself, or if you call ahead for me?

**Which hospital do you recommend?** Why? Would you take your own family there? How is that hospital rated?

**Is my insurance company a good one**? What problems might I have using this insurance? Do you have any suggestions for getting better care from my insurance company, or do you think I should get a different insurance plan? Do I need a social worker to help me?

**What vaccinations do I need?** Do you have a schedule of my revaccination times?

**Considering my family history, what are my highest-risk illnesses? How can I prevent them? How can I detect them earlier?**

Do I have habits I should change? Do you have treatments that can help me change them?

What vitamins and nutrients should I take?

**How often do I need regular checkups?** Do you remind me through the office, or is it my responsibility to initiate scheduling?

What should I keep in my medicine cabinet? What first-aid book do you recommend?

Should I take Heimlich and CPR training? Where? When? Should my spouse/significant other and family learn these techniques? Do I need to take CPR training for infants or children, or for my grandchildren?

Do I need a disease bracelet? Do I need a wallet card?

**In case of a disaster like Hurricane Katrina, whom do I call?** If you don't know, whom do you suggest I contact who could give me more information?

## Office Operations

**Can you provide a list of all office staff with whom I may need to talk?** (This list should cover doctors, nurses, medical assistants, aides, lab personnel, technicians, social workers, receptionists, billing clerks, insurance liaison personnel, office manager, and patient-relations manager.)

If I need to change an appointment, whom do I call? If I need an emergency appointment, whom do I call?

If I have a problem getting a test performed, whom do I call?

If have an insurance problem, whom do I call?

How much time do you schedule for an appointment? How do I obtain a longer visit if I need one? Are you usually on time, or do you usually run late? What things can I do to help you see me more efficiently? How can I find out if you are running late and whether I should come later than scheduled?

Do you have a standard family history form?

Do you have a standard review-of-systems form? Should I complete it before I come for a visit? Should I send it to the office before I come, so if I need more time or more tests you can arrange for them?

Do you have standard forms for medication, prior illnesses, diagnoses, and other physicians?

If I have questions about a new treatment for my condition that I read about on the Internet or in the newspaper, how do I let you know?

May I keep my own personal "home medical record"? Can the office give me copies of my reports and your notes to put into my record if I need them?

Do you have privacy rules and regulations? May I have a copy?

Do you have general information brochures or guidelines for your patients?

**Can I record what you tell me about my health and your recommendations, so my family and I can listen to it again at home?**

## Communicating with the Office

**If I have questions about my symptoms or treatment, whom do I call in the office during business hours?** Whom do I call after hours? Who covers your practice if you are not available? Will you call me back with answers to my questions?

Will the office call me to give me test results? If not, when do I call in to get the results?

Can I have a copy of my medical record?

## If You Have an Illness, Injury, or Disease: Questions about Treatment

### Making the Diagnosis and Choosing Treatment

**Why do I have these symptoms?** (Provide doctor with a symptom list.)

Will the treatments cure my condition or only make it better? What are the benefits? **What are the side effects?** Can I take these medicines with all my other pills? Can I take them with food? What do I do if I miss a dose?

How long will it take for the treatments to work? If they have not worked by then, what should I do?

**Are there any special dietary requirements or restrictions with my condition?** Should I take vitamins? Should I exercise? Can I travel? Is having intercourse okay? Will I benefit from rehabilitation?

How long have I had my condition? What caused it?

Which over-the-counter medications should I take for my disease, and which should I avoid? Are there complementary or alternative therapies for my disease, and do they work?

Are there clinical trials or experimental treatments for my disease? Do you participate in any of them? Where can I find out about them? Where can I get them? Would such treatments be good for me?

### Certainty of the Diagnosis

Do I need a second opinion by another pathologist about my diagnosis? Can you send my X-rays or scans to another radiologist for a second opinion? Can you advise me how to arrange for the second opinion by a radiologist or pathologist? How quickly can it be done?

**Are there specialists I should see regarding my diagnosis, treatment, or rehabilitation?**

## Prognosis and Getting More Information
**If you had this disease, what would you do?**

Once my disease is better, could it come back? If so, when? What is the first sign of it returning? Can tests monitor if it is returning?

Do you have any written information or pamphlets for me about my illness (or injury or disease)?

Is there a patient support group for my condition? Is there a nonprofit organization that deals with my disease (like the American Cancer Society or the American Heart Association)?

**Is there an Internet site or toll-free number where I can get further information about my illness?**

What should I tell my family about my disease? Can they catch it? Is it inherited? Can it be prevented?

It will be useful to review this list of questions periodically as a guide for issues that have not been covered by your physician or the staff. The quality of your medical care will be improved by your revisiting some of these issues with your primary doctor and any specialists or consultants. If your doctor has provided only incomplete answers to some of these questions, you might need further specialist consultations.

### Tips

- Write down every question you can think of, and bring the list with you. Also bring a family member or friend, if possible.
- Ask every question on your list.
- Make sure your doctor is listening. If he is distracted (typing, writing, reading), ask your question again.
- Listen to and remember each answer. Record it. Think about it. If you're puzzled, tell the doctor why—and do it now.
- Ask all follow-up questions now, not at a later visit.

## Contemporary Medicine and Communicating with Your Doctor

Regardless of the shape future health-care reform takes, more patients will be insured and in need of care. The result: your doctor will have a busier practice. You will have less time to get the answers you need to stay healthy, recover from illness, or get the best care for your disease or condition. Asking these questions, or all of them that apply to you, will get you the more comprehensive attention you need—and far better care.

Heavily managed-care programs like HMOs, ACOs, or some PPOs may not authorize many treatments unless you push for them. Asking all the right questions will encourage your doctor to go to bat for you, to get you the care you really need. Doctors and nurses may not pay attention to all these important issues with patients who are passive and don't ask questions, but by bringing your list of important questions and issues and being insistent about getting potentially lifesaving advice, you can overcome the superficial, rushed care so often associated with today's medicine.

All health-care reforms will ultimately require your doctor to add an electronic medical record, and this change can benefit you. By accessing your lab and X-ray results and any notes from your doctor visits and consultations, you can read how you are doing and ask questions about anything you don't understand. When you pay attention and ask the right questions, you become a savvier consumer of medical care—and that is exactly what our national leaders want you to become. That's today's medical care: it's better for you, but there's more for you to do.

All the changes in medical care make it more likely that your care will be moved to other doctors or care networks, so you must be certain that the transfer of your care is efficient and complete. Make sure your records and results are transferred to and understood by your new physicians and their offices; ask your new doctors if they have all your records, have reviewed them, and know what else needs to be done. Since things can be lost or misplaced, keep copies of your medical records and bring them with you to your first visit. And the question you must always ask is, "Have you seen all my records? If not, here they are!"

# Chapter 12

# You Have Only One Body—
# Better Take Care of It!

Have you heard any stories like this? Ben was fifty-three and a former smoker. I saw him for a newly diagnosed lung cancer. "Well, doc," he said, "I smoked one or two packs a day all my life since I was just a kid, maybe thirteen. But you know, I got smart—ever since they found this tumor on my lung. Now I've stopped smoking completely. My family doctor, she did try to get me to quit a couple of times, but when I tried to stop, it only lasted about a week. She finally gave up and just accepted that I was always going to smoke. My wife kept on nagging me to stop until I yelled at her that I just couldn't do it—but now I guess I proved I can."

Ben was sincere about how proud he was that he had finally stopped smoking, but unfortunately, his cancer had already spread to his lymph nodes and bones, and it would be impossible to cure him; he died eight months after his diagnosis, and eight months after quitting smoking. He had stopped smoking too late … by about forty years. Tragically, Ben knew that his smoking would prevent him from seeing his grandchildren grow up.

It's sad that although we have many more medicines and support groups to help patients kick their bad health habits, like smoking, drinking, or not exercising, very few patients ever ask their primary doctors to help them quit. And all too often, the patients' family members just give up trying to helping them. Like Ben, people with bad habits are just living on borrowed time until heart disease, lung problems, or even cancer catches up with them.

The topic may seem to be too superficial for *Surviving American Medicine*, but that fact is, doctors need to be giving this sort of pep talk more often. The reminder may just help save a few more lives … maybe even yours. Unfortunately, there are too few pep talks, really sincere advice, in medicine today—a result of too many patients, too little time. So be sure you ask your doctor for help.

## Committing Yourself to Health

You can't replace your body. Do you schedule regular health checkups? Do you keep the appointments with your physician? Do you eat a healthy diet? Do you put toxic things into your body (like cigarette smoke, excessive alcohol, or illegal drugs)? Do you ask your doctor about changes you can make to improve your lifestyle?

Being healthy and happy for your full lifetime requires serious commitment. This chapter is very short, but in some ways it is the most important one. You must find the inner resources and external influences that will motivate you to follow any medical advice you're given and to care for your body in a comprehensive, consistent, and prompt manner. The consequences of neglect are suffering, frustration, and untimely and preventable disability.

Behavioral changes are tough. To help make them stick, consider writing down your resolutions (it does not have to be on New Year's) and posting them on your refrigerator or desk. Discuss them with your spouse, family, and friends; let them know that your commitment is real and that you need their help, even if it seems like it isn't working at first. Pick a day to start your new, healthier lifestyle. Challenge another friend with similar habits to a contest to see who can overcome them most successfully. Join a support group or social network to help make the resolutions stick. Record your progress each day, on paper or a computer or smart phone. Consider getting an app to help encourage you to stick it out.

If your spouse, relative, or friend is neglecting his health, you can help by encouraging him to see a physician and supporting him when he keeps the appointment. Fulfilling your role as his loving family member or true friend also includes a moral responsibility to help him find good health care and use it effectively. That means urging him to keep his appointments, take his prescribed medicine, and not neglect any symptoms.

To ensure you have the right plan for preserving your health, maintain some type of health insurance at all times. Meet with your primary-care doctor annually to get a checkup and review your diet, your habits, your stress level, and your weight. Make sure you get answers to every question you have—advice about preventive care that will help you maintain your health. If you are having trouble making a change (like stopping smoking, following a healthier diet, exercising, or losing weight), insist that the doctor help you do better. Many medicines and physical interventions, such as support groups, exercise, or yoga, can help make the difference between success and a longer life, and failure, illness, and even death.

Over the past few years, employers have begun to realize the financial benefits of having healthy employees, and many businesses have initiated incentive programs offering lower insurance costs to employees who improve their weight or blood pressure or stop smoking. This is a formal added encouragement to help people be healthier, happier—and more effective workers. If your employer asks if you would like such a program, sign on. If your employer does not ask, talk to your human-resources department (or your boss) to see if one can be started. These programs are very effective.

## Crisis Management

In addition to diligently following your doctor's advice about health maintenance, promise yourself that you will take care of any potential problem rapidly and urgently. Work and shopping can wait. If a new symptom or condition arises, see your doctor immediately.

If you are in an accident and seriously injured, things sometimes take care of themselves—an ambulance arrives and speeds you off to the nearest trauma center. But too many people wave off the ambulance, saying, "No, I'm okay. I'll just see the doc later." Don't make that error. Go to the emergency room and let the hospital staff check you for hidden injuries that can only be detected by X-rays and tests.

If you develop severe pain, bleeding, shortness of breath, dizziness, or any other frightening or serious problem, call your doctor at once and either go to her office or to whatever ER she recommends. What if your doctor is not on call to answer your question? Go to the ER anyway, and let the hospital locate her; they're usually much better at that than you are. But don't stay home or at the office and just "let things pass." Too many people die that way.

What if you don't have insurance but you have serious symptoms? Living—and figuring out your bills later—is much better than dying or suffering incapacitating or permanent complications. So go immediately to an ER for evaluation.

## Tips

- Promise yourself good health.
- Use every trick to motivate yourself to keep good health habits.
- Request and follow your doctor's advice.
- Ask family and friends for their support and encouragement.

## Today's Medicine and Your Commitment to Health

Although changes in health-care are providing new insurance vehicles for obtaining care, new websites to help you access that care, and more inclusive coverage for preventive care, there is no substitute for your commitment to seeing a doctor regularly for checkups and to get symptoms addressed. That's a personal decision only you can make.

You can expect health-insurance plans to start giving you incentives, like lower premiums and costs, for maintaining healthy habits and an appropriate weight. Look for plans with these incentives. Not only will they save you money, but they will help you live longer.

# Chapter 13

# Keeping Track of Your Medical Care: Your Medical Record and Scorecard

In life, knowing where you are, where you've been, and where you're going is important in accomplishing any goal. The same is true in medicine: knowing these three things is critical in protecting your health and the health of your family. Patients tend to think that keeping track of their medical care is solely the responsibility of their physician, but that's just not so anymore. With the greater stress and pressure in physicians' offices and the increasing volume of documentation and consent forms, it has become harder for medical offices and hospitals to be aware of a patient's past history and current treatments and problems. If your doctors and nurses have overlooked an important fact in your medical history, they can make a dangerous error! How can you make sure your health-care team is up-to-date?

## Your Personal Medical Record

In other areas of life, you keep detailed records. When you file your tax return each year, you keep a copy. You keep records of your insurance policies and claims. You hang on to warrantees, receipts, diplomas, and even pictures and letters.

It's remarkable how few people keep track of their personal medical records in a similar fashion. Why is this important? Granted, in many circumstances, it's unnecessary, because you may remain with the same doctor for most your life, and if you change doctors, your former physician should send copies of all your records to your new doctor.

But often life is far more complicated: we move, our doctors retire, our health-insurance plan changes, we take a new job with different insurance, or our hospitals change. Physicians often pass away before their patients do. Hospitals disappear as a result of mergers and bankruptcies. Emergencies— hurricanes, earthquakes, even a fire in your doctor's office—can prevent you from having access to your medical records. For example, one of my patients had her ovaries removed twenty years ago. Because she had not kept copies of her medical records, I tried to get them through the doctors and hospital that had cared for her. The hospital had gone bankrupt; their records were lost. The doctor had died, and no one knew where his records had gone. So to this day, we do not know what illness she had, whether it will influence her risk of certain future illnesses (like breast cancer), or what possible genetic changes she might have transmitted to her children. So keep your own records, in your house.

Having your own personal medical record—with your complete history and a good description of your illness—helps ensure that when you go to another medical office or hospital, the nurses, physicians, and other health-care personnel can make accurate diagnoses. None of us wants our doctors to make errors in taking care of us.

When my patients bring in their own medical records, I always use them to be certain I have all the information necessary to care for those patients. If you keep your personal record, your doctors may never need to use it, but usually it will be helpful at least a few times. If your doctor needs it even once, it is well worth the small amount of time you have spent in starting the record and keeping it current. And it's always good security to have your health summary with you when you travel with you, in the event that you have to go to an emergency room.

In appendix 1, I have outlined all the important elements of a personal medical record. Although it seems like a long list, once you have filled out the forms initially, most of the record never needs to be changed again. Each section may have to be regularly updated slightly, and that small amount of time will help keep your patient medical record comprehensive.

Your physician's office should help you by providing almost all the data. Ask for the office's demographic page, which can serve as the basis for the first section in your record. Also ask for copies of any of your surgical notes, pathology reports, histories and physicals, and discharge summaries. Some offices may charge up to twenty-five cents a page for some records, and a radiology department might charge several dollars for each CD of important X-rays which you could someday need, but often they can provide you with a free or low-cost CD of X-rays. Whatever the cost, it's a small price to pay to keep your personal medical records as comprehensive as possible.

## How Good a Patient Are You?

I've talked a lot about how to evaluate your doctor and your health care. But there's another important aspect of your medical care that merits evaluation—you. Are you a good patient? Are you taking all the steps necessary to stay healthy and prevent disease? Now it's time to complete your own scorecard. The following self-assessment can tell you whether you need some help from your family or your doctor to become a better patient or take preventive action, and thereby get better health.

I've designed the scorecards in this book to help you rate yourself and your wellness care. They are based on my many years of experience, not on statistics. But they will be useful as you try to determine whether you are as good a patient as you need to be in order to live a long and happy life. So take the test below and see how you do. If you don't score as well as you would like, discuss it with your doctor to see how he can help you improve.

## Good Patient Scorecard

**Answer the following questions, giving yourself one point for each "yes" answer and zero points for each "no":**

1. I have a primary doctor, and I have seen him in the past twelve months.

2. I have my next appointment with my physician scheduled on my calendar.
3. I go to my doctor appointment with a list of questions and concerns.
4. I take my spouse, family, friend, or advocate with me to my appointment, or I record information during my doctor visit on paper, smart phone, or tape recorder.
5. I have asked my doctor about all the following: diet; weight; exercise; risk of diseases (heart disease, cancer, diabetes, lung disease); PPD skin test for tuberculosis; unhealthy habits (smoking, drinking, illicit drugs); screening for cancer; vitamins and nutrients.
6. I know the names of my doctor's nurse, receptionist, and billing clerk, and I understand whom to call and how to contact the office for any problem.
7. All my vaccinations are up-to-date. For adults, those include tetanus, flu, pneumococcal pneumonia, and sometimes shingles vaccine (and HPV, for women). For children, those include tetanus-diphtheria-pertussis, measles-mumps-rubella, varicella chicken pox, polio, hemophilus influenza, and hepatitis A and B.
8. I know my blood pressure, cholesterol, and fasting blood sugar.
9. I have health insurance and keep the card in my wallet or purse.
10. I have a wallet card or digital chip with my doctor's name, phone number, insurance number, medications, and emergency contacts.
11. I keep copies of my medical records.
12. I discuss unhealthy habits with my doctor as appropriate: lack of exercise, smoking, drinking, drug abuse, unsafe sex, excess eating or obesity, depression.
13. Cancer screening by gender:
    a. Women: I have had a Pap smear and HPV test for cervical cancer, and if I'm over forty, I've had a mammogram for breast cancer.
    b. Men: If I'm over forty, I've have had a prostate examination, and if I'm over forty or fifty, I've discussed with my doctor a PSA screening for prostate cancer.

    c.   Both genders: I have had a skin exam for melanoma and a mouth exam for oral cancer. If I'm over fifty, I've had a colonoscopy or sigmoidoscopy for colon cancer. If I'm a current or former smoker, I've had a chest CT scan for lung cancer.

14.  I know which hospital I will use in an emergency and where the ER is located.

15.  I have a durable power of attorney for health care, a living will, and a signed advanced directives form (an order indicating "fully resuscitate" or "do not resuscitate," as desired).

Scoring: Your goal is 15 points.

0 to 11: Poor—you need to focus on and improve your health care.

12 or 13: Good

14 or 15: Excellent

## Are You and Your Doctor Preventing Disease?

Not only is it important to be a good patient, as you evaluated above, but it's also vital that you and your physicians commit to preventing disease before it strikes. Take the following test to determine your disease-prevention score.

## Disease-Prevention Scorecard

**Answer the following questions, giving yourself one point for each "yes" answer and zero points for each "no":**

1.  My blood pressure is less than 140 systolic and less than 90 diastolic (under 140/90).
2.  My cholesterol is less than 200.
3.  My fasting blood sugar is less than 110.
4.  I don't smoke or abuse drugs.
5.  I drink two or fewer drinks per day.
6.  I exercise an average of fifteen minutes per day or more.

7. My vaccinations are up to date: flu (annually), pneumonia (every five years), HPV (women over ten and under twenty-six), and tetanus (every ten years).
8. My weight is okay—body mass index (BMI) less than 25. (To calculate BMI, go online to NHLBISupport.com/bmi/.)
9. My diet includes all of the following: five helpings or more of fruits or vegetables per day; red meat less than twice per week; fish at least twice per week; mostly low-fat and low trans-fat foods; nuts; olive oil; whole grains.
10. I take aspirin daily, or I have discussed it with my physician.
11. I have been checked for the following: hepatitis C; HIV (as appropriate); bone density (anyone over fifty); PPD; colonoscopy or sigmoidoscopy and annual stool occult blood test (over fifty); mammogram (women over forty or fifty); Pap smear and HPV (women over fifteen); prostate exam (men over forty); annual PSA (men over forty to fifty), or discussed PSA with my doctor.
12. I have had an eye exam in the last two years.
13. I have had an annual physical exam in the last year.
14. I have had the screening blood tests my doctor recommends. (Recommended screenings usually include a complete blood count CBC, complete metabolic panel CMP, iron level, B12 level, fasting lipid panel, and thyroid test.)
15. If I'm over fifty, I have had a carotid ultrasound and a whole-body CT scan or ultrasound (for aneurysms).
16. I have an emergency evacuation plan for myself and my family.
17. I have had home-safety education and discussed it with my family.

Scoring: Your goal is 17.

0 to 12: Poor—discuss with your physician.

13 to 15: Good

16 to 17: Excellent

## Tips

- Keep copies of your medical records and take them to your health-care visits. Use your doctor's office to help you create a comprehensive medical history.
- Assess whether you are a good patient. If you're not, ask your doctor for help.
- Work with your doctor to focus on preventive medicine.

## Contemporary Medicine, Medical Scorecards, and Personal Records

Personal responsibility is a key component of health-care reform. The scorecards being promoted by government regulations and private insurance plans will give you information about doctors and hospitals, so use these tools to gain more confidence in your care.

In fact, new changes to health care will help you take personal responsibility. The increased use of electronic health records makes it easier to get more complete, readable medical records, as well as copies of laboratory results and radiology reports. All of this makes it easier to keep and understand your personal health records.

With more ways to get medical coverage and more variety in health-care programs, there's an increased likelihood that you will change your health insurance and your physicians. If that happens, having your own personal health records will facilitate getting prompter, more complete, and more accurate medical care.

# Chapter 14

# Dealing with Minor Medical Problems: Medication under Your Doctor's Guidance

When you feel ill, your first thought is almost always, *What can I do to get better?* You'll probably have over-the-counter medications on hand, but sometimes your doctor would like you to have some prescription medications at home to take when the medical office is closed. Other countries don't require prescriptions for commonly used antibiotics, but that's not the case in the United States. So should you have those or other drugs on hand in your house?

Medicines comprise an important part of your medical care, because they bridge wellness and more serious symptoms requiring an office visit, urgent care, or emergency-room evaluation. By discussing the topic ahead of time with your doctor, you will know what medicines to have on hand in case of mild illness.

Your medicine cabinet is important in keeping you healthy, because often symptoms arise when pharmacies are closed, and prompt treatment with the right medicine can help you avoid unnecessary suffering. Except in cases of the most urgent medical illnesses, such as trauma, chest pain, or cardiac arrest, emergency-room care is slow and inefficient. So maintaining a supply of medications and using them as your doctor has recommended can prevent a long (and possibly unnecessary) visit to the hospital. Keeping your medicine cabinet filled, and knowing how to use your prescriptions correctly, are important survival skills.

One of my patients could have avoided a hospital stay costing $50,000. Because he had a low white blood cell count that put him at risk of infection, I had prescribed antibiotics for him to keep on hand, telling him that if he developed a high fever to take them immediately and call my office. When he developed a high fever and cough—it was probably pneumonia—he ignored my advice and decided to let the illness run its course. He finally called me when he grew very short of breath. It was late at night, and he had never bothered to fill the prescription. Since his symptoms had worsened so badly in the absence of any antibiotics, he ended up in the hospital for ten days. And he could have avoided everything—the severe pneumonia and shortness of breath, the hospitalization, the very high co-payment for the hospital stay—just by keeping the appropriate medicines on hand at home.

So make it a point to ask your doctor, "What emergency medicines do you want me to have, and how do you want me to use them? Do you have an instruction sheet, or will your nurse give me some guidance?"

## Medicines You Should Have in Your Home

Although I am not going to recommend specific medicines for your medicine cabinet—that's for you to discuss with your physician—I will tell you which *types* of medicines you should discuss with your doctor. After reviewing your illnesses, your physician will determine which medicines are safe and teach you how and when to take them. You can get more information about them from your nurses and pharmacist.

Take the following list with you to discuss with your physician. Expect clear, specific answers about each type of medicine.

- **vitamins:** multivitamin, folic acid, B6, B12, C, D, or others
- **nutrients:** calcium, iron, glucosamine, fish oil, Coenzyme Q, or others
- **aspirin**
- **pain medicines:** aspirin, acetaminophen, ibuprofen or equivalent, or others

- **sinus and throat medicine:** oral decongestants, nasal decongestant sprays, nasal steroid sprays, cough syrup, cough drops, or others
- **anti-allergy medicines:** diphenhydramine, loratidine or equivalent, epinephrine auto-injectors, corticosteroids, or others
- **antibiotics:** respiratory antibiotics, urinary antibiotics, or others
- **bronchitis/asthma medicines:** bronchodilator inhalers, steroid inhalers, antibiotics, or others
- **stomach medicines:** antacids, cimetidine or equivalent, omeprazole or equivalent, Pepto-Bismol, antiemetics, simethicone, or others
- **colon medicines:** stool softeners, Milk of Magnesia, suppositories, loperamide or equivalent, fiber, or others
- **ointments:** corticosteroid ointment, antibiotic ointment, antifungal ointment, pain ointment (Solarcaine or equivalent), or others
- **first-aid supplies:** bandages, tape, gauze pads, antiseptics, or others
- **special products:** thermometer, automatic blood pressure monitor, glucose monitor, weight scale, or others

## Medicine Lists

You should always know what medicines you are taking and have that list with you in your wallet or purse. You never know when an emergency will occur and that list will help first responders or emergency-room personnel treat you properly. Attach a list of your medicines and illnesses to your refrigerator, either outside on the door or inside on the first shelf in the door, for emergency purposes; paramedics know to look there for medication lists. Share that information with your family and friends as well.

## You and Your Pharmacist

Many people are turning to mail-order sources to save on the cost of medicine. But keep in mind that you receive valuable information from your own dedicated neighborhood pharmacists, who usually can provide detailed advice on potentially dangerous drug side effects, dangerous drug combinations, or how and when to take medicines. Such personalized advice might be impossible to find if you use mail-order sources for your medicines. In fact, pharmacists came in first in a national poll in which people were asked, "Whom do you trust the most?" (Ministers came in second, and doctors third.) So essential is your pharmacist's advice that you should always ask her any questions about any of your medications, whether it's a brand-new prescription or a medicine you've been taking for years. Here are some of the most important questions to ask:

- What are all the side effects of this medicine? When should I take it? Do I take it with or without food? Can I drink alcohol with this medicine?
- Here is a list of my allergies. Do they interact with this new medicine? Here is a list of my current medicines. Are there any interactions with this new drug?
- Can I take my usual over-the-counter medicines and vitamins with this drug?
- Do I need any tests from my doctor to monitor this new medicine? Are there long-term side effects if I take this medicine for many months? When should I visit my doctor to look for any of these side effects?
- If I begin to have difficulty affording this medicine, does the pharmaceutical company have a special discount program?
- Are there any package inserts with information for patients? Do you have a printed information sheet on this medicine?

In addition to the pharmacist, other resources are available to help you manage and monitor your own medicines. Your physician should provide a good understanding of any drug you're taking and its side effects, and he should advise you when to call him for side effect symptoms. The office nurse can give similar recommendations and may be able to provide you with an information sheet. Information about most medicines is available online at Drugs.com, or you can purchase a *Physicians' Desk Reference* or obtain short summaries online at PDR.net to read about each of your medicines. Much of the description in the *PDR* is very complex and difficult to understand, but the information on side effects and adverse events can be very useful.

## Tips

- Know how your doctor wants you to treat minor medical problems.
- Ask your primary-care physician which medications you should keep in your medicine cabinet for infection (antibiotics), chest pain (nitrates, aspirin), diarrhea, nausea, or pain.
- If children are ever in your house, be certain all your medicines have childproof lids.

## Contemporary Health Care and Medications

With health-care reforms, physicians will be stressing coordinated care for chronic illnesses. Coordinators (usually nurse practitioners) will make sure you have more medications on hand to avoid unnecessary emergency care or doctor visits. In general, patients will be expected to take more responsibility for their own health care.

There also will be increased restrictions on which medications will be covered by insurance, and a similarly increased reliance on over-the-counter medicines. Many drugs that currently require a prescription will become nonprescription medicines, just as omeprazole and loratidine have done in the past. For you, this means increased availability but also increased costs, as most insurance doesn't cover over-the-counter medicines. So you should discuss with your physicians and nurses which drugs you should keep on hand, and which ones are available as less expensive generics.

# Section 2:
# Dealing with Disease and Serious Illness

# Chapter 15

## Second Opinions

The most valuable quality-control tool in getting outstanding medical care is the second opinion. To be wholly confident in dealing with any serious, chronic, or life-threatening disease, you must make sure that any decisions about the nature of the disease and its treatment are correct. This chapter will help you know when, where, and how to get a second opinion (or a third, fourth, or fifth).

Are you seeing the right doctor? Is there something missing in your care? Do you have the wrong diagnosis? Do you really trust what your doctor told you? Are you not getting better? Often a second opinion is the only way to answer those questions and improve your health care.

After receiving a diagnosis of incurable lung cancer (non-small cell type), a forty-nine-year-old woman came to see me for a second opinion. When I had her pathology slides reviewed and special immuno-histochemistry stains performed to confirm the diagnosis, the diagnosis changed: she actually was suffering from a mediastinal germ cell tumor, curable with chemotherapy. She received the appropriate drugs and remains in remission today. The moral of this story: if you are told you have an incurable disease, get a second opinion. Don't worry about offending your doctor; he would do the same thing in your position. Second opinions are common practice, and your doctor will understand. If he doesn't, he probably is not the right doctor for you.

There is a certain psychology involved in receiving a medical opinion. Certainly any patient wants to be told, "Everything is okay—I can't find anything wrong." This is reassuring, but especially if symptoms persist or abnormal lab findings are unexplained, patients still have the nagging feeling that something serious might be wrong. And if a patient is told, "You have a serious disease," he wants to be sure that the grim diagnosis isn't a mistake. In either case, the patient always wants only good news, and second opinions can help.

Even if the original diagnosis of a serious condition was made at a well-known hospital by well-regarded doctors, you should still get a second opinion. Even the best doctors make mistakes.

There are several methods that doctors, medical centers, and hospitals use to prevent errors in diagnosis. Those include consultations with other doctors; a review of pathology opinions among several pathologists; informal conferences (daily discussions among the doctors in a clinic or practice to review all new patients, hospital patients, and problem situations); formal conferences (such as cardiac catheterization conferences or breast cancer clinic patient presentations); tumor board presentations (in which pathologists, surgeons, and radiation and medical oncologists discuss cancer patients and make suggestions about diagnosis and treatment); and multidisciplinary hospital rounds. If you have been diagnosed with a serious condition, be certain your doctor has used some of these methods to verify your diagnosis and select the best therapy for you.

Another patient who came to me for a second opinion was a fifty-one-year-old woman who had felt a lump in her breast. Her surgeon, an internationally respected breast cancer specialist, could not feel what she felt, and her mammogram was normal. After receiving that news and being told to come back in a year, the patient was happy and reassured. But she still felt the lump. It got bigger, she worried more, and after twelve months she came to me for a second opinion. By that time I could feel the lump too. It was biopsied and found to be invasive cancer. Unfortunately, scans revealed that she had developed bone metastases and was no longer curable. The lesson: since mammograms miss 15 percent of breast cancers, the surgeon should have done more studies and more exams to find the mass earlier, when it might have been cured. And since she remained increasingly suspicious that the lump was not getting better, the patient should have sought a second opinion as soon as she realized her symptoms were not improving, not a year later when the cancer had become widespread and fatal.

Although nearly everyone has heard stories about how a second opinion has helped improve someone's quality of care, most patients are very reluctant to ask for a second opinion. At the heart of this reluctance is their fear that if they do, their doctor won't like them anymore or will refuse to see them again.

How do second opinions help you?

No matter who your doctor is, no matter where your doctor works (whether a community clinic or a university), he can make errors, overlooking important diagnoses or tests that could help him cure a disease before it worsens to become incurable or even terminal. How can you know when to ask your doctor to reevaluate? How can you know when to seek a second opinion? And how can you gain the courage and confidence to get a second opinion without fearing the wrath of your physician and his staff?

One method is to ask, "You know, doctor, I still have these symptoms, and I wonder if you could reevaluate them. If you can't find out what's going on, maybe we can get a second opinion from another doctor who can help us work this out together." Or you can try a more straightforward approach: "I know you've done all you can for me, but I really think we need to get a second opinion. Whom should I see so that we can continue to make progress in my illness?"

If your doctor threatens not to keep you as a patient if you get a second opinion, then you're probably seeing the wrong physician. Although most doctors accept the need for second opinions, some won't consider sending you to another specialist. This can occur because they are overconfident (they think they are experts who know everything); they fear losing you to another doctor; or they are embarrassed because they are uncertain and fear a second opinion will reveal their deficiencies. Regardless of the reason for the reluctance, you are at risk of having inappropriate diagnosis or care, and you could be losing the opportunity to cure or control your condition.

Remember, you always have the right to a second opinion. You do not need your doctor's permission to get one.

Often a physician will obtain informal second opinions on your behalf. For example, I was caring for a fifty-year-old woman who had a very small breast cancer. Because she had gotten regular mammograms, the radiologists were able to pick up a very tiny breast cancer, less than a third of an inch in diameter. Because it was so small, I felt that this tumor did not require any additional chemotherapy, just radiation and hormone treatments. I told the patient that in order to confirm my impression, I wanted to contact the doctors who were conducting international trials in the management of very small breast cancers. I telephoned three leading cancer researchers, all of whom agreed that no chemotherapy was necessary. The second, third, and fourth opinions that I had obtained informally for my patient made her more confident in my care, saved her the time and expense of traveling to other cities, and resulted in an effective, less toxic type of treatment. If you feel that your doctor needs more help in planning your treatment, ask him to consult other specialists about your condition.

If you have symptoms that persist for over a week, or that worsen despite treatment, go back to your doctor for more testing and a new diagnosis. Never accept suggestions over the phone without a repeat exam by the doctor; only she can give you the attention you need. If she cannot make a diagnosis and just wants to watch your tests, get a second opinion. Remember, you can't trade in your body for a new model. Insist on first-class care, or get a second opinion from a doctor who will give you the quality care you deserve.

## Types of Second Opinions

**Diagnostic Review:** The first type of second opinion is the one intended to confirm a diagnosis or finding. For example, a biopsy that shows cancer can be referred to another pathologist at another institution to verify the diagnosis. Your own doctor can arrange this second opinion for you; you don't have to be seen by anyone else. Just ask your doctor to request that the pathologist send out the biopsy for another opinion. (This may require authorization by your insurance, but they rarely refuse.) Also, an abnormal finding on your X-ray or CT scan can be reviewed by another radiologist. Again, just ask your doctor to request that the radiology department obtain a second evaluation of the results.

**Evaluation and Management:** Another type of second opinion would help ascertain whether your specialist has made the correct diagnosis, evaluation, and plan for therapy. The doctor who provides this second opinion should also specialize in your illness or condition, and you should request this referral from your primary physician. If you have chronic low back pain, for example, an orthopedic surgeon's recommendation of surgery may be incorrect, and a second orthopedic specialist may determine that equal results can be achieved through medical management. (The first specialist's recommendation also may be perfectly correct, but in either case, you'll be reassured by a second opinion.) Insurance companies rarely decline a request for a second opinion in these situations, although most (other than PPOs and Medicare) are more reluctant to approve third or more opinions. (Your primary-care physician can help you get these approved.)

**Choice of Surgeon:** Another type of second opinion will help you choose the correct surgeon for an operation. If you are told you need surgery, it is wise to get a second opinion from another surgeon. When you go for that second opinion, ask the following important questions:

- Is the surgery necessary?
- Is the diagnosis correct?
- Which surgery is best?
- How high is the complication rate, in your experience?
- Which hospital is best?
- Which anesthesiologist is best?
- Will you do the surgery yourself, or will it be performed by an assistant, resident, fellow, or intern?
- How long will I be hospitalized?
- What are the possible complications?
- How many of these operations do you do every year?

## Have You Already Had a Second Opinion?

Since many good physicians routinely obtain informal second opinions on behalf of their patients, ask your doctor, "Have you discussed my case with other doctors?" Ideally, you will find out that your doctor has already asked the pathologist to review your test results with other pathologists in the same hospital or other medical centers. Or perhaps the radiologist has already reviewed your abnormal X-ray with others in her radiology group.

Your doctor may have even presented your case to other physicians in other specialties without your requesting it, in order to confirm the diagnosis or to select the best treatment. Or he may have presented a description of your illness at a tumor board or hospital conference and received the advice of other specialists to confirm the best treatment plan for you. And it would not be unusual for him to have called other national or regional experts on your behalf, before starting any tests or therapy.

Therefore, discuss these possibilities with your primary physician or specialists to be certain you really need a second opinion. This can increase your confidence in the care your current doctors are giving you and reassure you that a second opinion is not needed.

### The Ten Commandments of Second Opinions

I believe there are ten circumstances in which you should consider asking your physician for further evaluation or a second opinion:

1. You have a symptom that doesn't get better, or you do not have a definite diagnosis.
2. A treatment you are receiving for a disease doesn't seem to be working; your doctor says the treatments aren't working and there isn't anything else to do; or your doctor suggests hospice.
3. The treatment you're receiving seems too toxic or has side effects that bother you, and your doctor does not change your treatment.
4. You're in a patient support group for your illness, and other patients with the same disease are getting different kinds of care, different treatments, or different tests, and your doctor cannot explain why you need the treatments you have been receiving.
5. Your doctor doesn't talk to you and answer all your questions.
6. Your doctor doesn't know about new treatments, state-of-the-art therapies, or clinical trials that might help you, or he will

not call other centers on your behalf to find out about other treatments.

7. Your doctor is getting upset with you or your family.
8. You do not trust your doctor.
9. Your insurance does not authorize a treatment or test that your doctor has recommended for you, and your doctor cannot or will not appeal the denial. (A second opinion doctor's report can be sent to the insurance company—or to your lawyer—to convince the insurance company to authorize what is needed.)
10. Your doctor has not talked with you about *prevention* of diseases (like heart disease or cancer) and ignores your request for preventive advice and care.

## Third—or More—Opinions

If the first and second opinions differ, which is correct? If the second opinion is from a source that is more highly regarded (a university, famous specialist, or well-known treatment center), then it is logical to trust that opinion. A friend of mine with lung cancer visited the two most prestigious cancer centers in the world—and received two markedly different recommendations. So whom should she trust? She obtained a third opinion to ensure she was proceeding with the right therapy.

Sometimes you need to go beyond the second opinion, to a third, fourth, or even more. Fran Drescher, who introduced this book, needed *nine* opinions before her uterine cancer was diagnosed—and she survived! Take a lesson from her: do not stop asking questions until your condition improves or a proper diagnosis is confirmed so your treatments can begin.

## Getting Your Records

After you've made an appointment to see another doctor, it's crucial to have all your prior records—as complete a medical history as possible—at the new physician's office before you go for your first visit. You don't want to hear, "I can't tell what's wrong with you until I've seen the results of your old tests, biopsies, X-rays, hospital stays, and prior doctors' evaluations." When that happens, it could take another two to four weeks until the new doctor reevaluates you, and by then the doctor will be less focused on your problems than he was at your first visit.

So take the time to request that copies of all your relevant records from each of your prior doctors and hospital admissions be sent to the new doctor as soon as possible. How do you make sure they get there? The best way is to take them yourself. You should personally carry them from the prior doctors' offices and hospitals to the new doctor's office—and while you're at it, make copies for yourself as well, to establish your personal medical record (see appendix 1). If you are already maintaining your record at home, just copy any old information and supplement it with the most recent additions from the doctors' offices.

## Getting a Second Opinion with an HMO

One of the most frequent problems with HMOs is patients' frustration with limits on authorized care, especially when you have failed to recover with the treatments that have been given. If this has happened to you, then you will need a second opinion. HMOs allow you to obtain a second opinion from a physician within your plan, and they often quickly approve requests for a second opinion. However, if you request a second opinion from a physician outside the health plan, it is often initially denied.

The first step in the solution is to ask your own HMO primary-care physician for a second opinion referral, either within or outside the HMO network. If this request is denied, appeal that decision with your HMO. Each HMO has a process for appeal, usually involving a written request. I also recommend an immediate phone call to the medical director's office *with* a follow-up letter referencing your appeal for a second opinion. Remember to keep a record of each phone call, including the name of the person to whom you spoke and the date and time of the conversation.

If the HMO still does not authorize a second opinion, you can always go outside the health plan and just pay out of pocket. This is often worthwhile, since the second-opinion physician may suggest more appropriate medical care, and she may write a letter regarding the medical necessity for that care. With a letter of medical necessity from an outside consultant or specialist, you'll often find that appropriate care within the HMO will be authorized. You may have paid extra money to get your HMO to approve your specialized treatments, but it's worth the expense to get the proper care.

If you go outside your HMO to obtain a second opinion and/or treatment that was originally denied, and if you have a good written record of your HMO's failure to authorize the outside consultation or care, you may still get reimbursed for those medical bills by submitting them to the HMO anyway. If the bills are not paid, consider having a lawyer write your HMO stating that you may file suit to receive reimbursement. Then present your complaint to the state office of insurance (or the state office that regulates your HMO—see the list in appendix 4), and see if that office will advocate on your behalf. If your HMO still does not pay for the outside second opinion, consider going to small claims court to initiate your own lawsuit against the HMO. Small claims court does not require a lawyer, and with the appropriate documentation of the medical necessity for that second opinion and related treatments, the court will usually—but not always—decide in the patient's favor. Keep in mind, however, that small claims courts have an upper limit of the amount for which you can sue.

## Second Opinions: University Hospital or Community Center?

For a second opinion, should you go to the local hospital, a large community center, or a university? It really depends on the doctor involved, his credentials, and what sort of help you will need in addition to his care.

Community hospitals usually do not offer all the state-of-the-art treatments available at a university hospital, and the better-known specialists are more often found at universities rather than in community hospitals. However, care at university hospitals can seem impersonal; one of my patients told me she felt like something in a factory rather than a patient with a life-threatening problem.

Some community hospitals have specialized centers of excellence, which provide outstanding services. Similarly, physicians in some medical practices focus on only a few diseases and have put into place a broad range of supportive tests and procedures that comprise the comprehensive care some patients need. And in university hospitals, there are often (but not always) disease centers that are at the forefront of medicine for a specific illness. To determine which center is right for you, ask questions of your doctors and specialists, and do your own research on the web.

Usually you can't go wrong with a university hospital center that specializes in your disease. But one of my patients with ovarian cancer went for a second opinion to a nationally recognized university cancer center, only to have the young consultant there focus solely on her laboratory studies, unaware of the very promising clinical trial available for her. *So if you go to a university center, beware of getting an opinion from a less experienced faculty member—seek out the more experienced specialist. (You can check out his or her credentials at the university website.)* Another of my patients went to a different university center for his prostate cancer, and although there was a proven, effective standard therapy available for him, he was pushed into a clinical trial of an unproven Phase I drug with no evidence of a good track record in treating prostate cancer. Ultimately the patient returned to standard treatments after his tumor progressed on the experimental trial. So be certain to ask about all the options for your care, whether in a university setting or a community center.

Sometimes getting the care you need requires traveling to another city, and I recommend making that effort to get the best second (or third or fourth) opinion available and get your health-care plan back on track. Making the right decision at the right time gives you the best chance of surviving.

## Tips

- Second opinions are often necessary. Don't worry about what your first doctor will think of you if you ask for one.
- Follow my ten commandments of second opinions to determine if you need one.
- Do not be concerned if you need a third opinion; many people do.
- Although university centers are usually the best site for a second opinion, a community center can be better for certain patients. Check out the doctor's credentials and reputation before deciding.

## Today's Medicine and Second Opinions

The changes that come with health-care reform will make it harder to get all the tests and treatments you may need. Medical directors and utilization review nurses and/or committees will slow and restrict access to many tests and procedures to save money. So it will be increasingly important for you to know how to get second opinions and how to take that advice and use it effectively with the doctors in your health plan. Use doctors, nurses, and advocates (family and friends) to find the best professional advice possible.

As more nurse practitioners and physicians' assistants help in your care, you will need to ask them to check with the supervising doctor to see if anything else needs to be done. Don't hesitate to ask if you suspect you are not getting all the care you need, if you are not getting better, or if you are not getting prevention advice.

Contemporary medicine has developed standards for treatment, so your doctor should know the national guidelines for tests and treatments for any disease. If he does not know these (or know where you can read them yourself), get a second opinion to find out what the standards are and whether your doctor has been following them in your case. Better to check and be reassured than find out later that your physician has messed up!

# Chapter 16

# Practice Guidelines

Medical "breakthroughs" and new treatments are constantly reported and promoted on television, in newspapers and magazines, and all over the Internet. When you or a family member who is suffering from an illness hears of treatments other patients have received, you get excited, your heart beats faster, and hope soars. It's quite natural for you to want to start or at least consider these breakthrough treatments immediately.

However, the frequent response by a physician is, "Well, there's no proof yet that this treatment will help you!" Why might your doctor say this?

- Often the doctor is aware of the requested treatment and knows that it would be ineffective for a particular patient, or possibly even dangerous. When this is the case, she won't recommend the drug because it will not help you.
- Unfortunately, sometimes a physician won't recommend a particular treatment because the insurance company won't cover it (they often call it "experimental"), has pressured the physician not to give it (it might be more expensive than other therapies), or has refused to authorize it. Under these circumstances, the physician is acting primarily on behalf of the insurance company. Find out if this is the situation, and then ask the doctor to appeal any refusal, or get a second opinion about whether the treatment will actually help you.

- Sometimes, the doctor just does not know enough about the treatment and wants to see published articles that constitute proof of the drug's positive effects. In this case, show the doctor any information you have about the treatment, ask him to check with his colleagues or experts, or get another opinion if he doesn't want to check it out for you. A second opinion is worth whatever time or money it takes to find out if the new therapy is for you.

- Even if a new drug is useful in treating a disease, often the timing isn't right for its use in a particular patient's case, and better treatments should be used first. Standard treatments (regardless of whether they are more or less costly) may have better results than the new drug and therefore might be the preferred drug for initial treatment (with the new drug considered a possible option for later treatment). If this is the case, usually your doctor will explain it to you. But if you are not convinced by her words or if you are suspicious (that she is uninformed about the drug or treatment, is unwilling to fight the insurance company to get you access to it, or doesn't know how to access it), get a second opinion from another specialist.

If you are faced with a serious illness for which initial reports suggest a certain treatment might be beneficial, and if your doctor feels that this treatment program offers you the best chance of recovery or survival, then you have to work with your doctor to try to get access to the treatment. In this situation, even if there is not absolute medical proof of the treatment's success rate, there already is some published data to suggest it would benefit you.

## Evidence-Based Medicine

Across the medical spectrum, and especially in this era of health-care reform and closer insurance company review of requested treatments, physicians, administrators, insurance companies, and medical directors are moving toward evidence-based medicine. What is this, and is it good for you?

*Evidence-based medicine* is the terminology for using published data that prove the benefit of any treatment, surgery, or drug for a specific patient group. For example, a particular drug might have been shown effective in medical studies reported in peer-reviewed journals—that is, journals in which other doctors or scientists review the study's findings, confirm that its results are valid, and deem the paper acceptable for publication. In that case, the authors of the published study have specified what type of patients the treatment has been shown to benefit.

National physician organizations have used these reported studies to develop *practice guidelines* for doctors to follow. (They may also be called "pathways" or "treatment templates.") Treatment authorizations by insurance companies or Medicare are based upon these practice guidelines and/or published results, so you can ask your doctor or try to find out on the Internet which practice guidelines apply to your condition. Your doctor or a disease organization (e.g., the American Cancer Society or the American Heart Association) can point you toward the correct website to find the guidelines.

It is very difficult for a patient to know when to argue with a physician to try to get a new therapy, especially after the physician has said, "There's just no evidence proving that this treatment will benefit you." When should you challenge this statement? When should you fight to obtain a treatment that you have heard about?

Physicians admit that much medical knowledge is still incomplete. Doctors follow the *standard of care*—in other words, the standard that most doctors in a community generally use based upon not only published articles, but also logical, scientifically rational applications of proven principles and the advice of experts (usually university professors). Still, you should ask your doctor, "Are there published guidelines for my disease? Where can I find them, or can you give me a copy?" You can also get a second opinion from a university expert in your disease; he or she can give you a letter to get a new treatment authorized by your insurance company.

Sometimes, even though a particular treatment might be beneficial, those who pay for the clinical care (e.g., insurance companies, HMOs, ACOs, Medicare, Medicaid, or even employers) have concluded that the cost of that treatment, compared to its benefits, is just too high. Many insurance programs, and even physicians, will refuse to consider such a test or treatment even if a patient might benefit from it. In the United States, public health-care economists usually use the *cost/benefit analysis* as a criterion for authorizing treatments. After determining the cost of a new treatment, they will review published reports of the survival of patients who have used it (compared to patients who haven't). Then they will calculate a ratio of the cost to the number of years of life "saved." The costlier treatments are not routinely approved, while the less costly ones are.

The current target cutoff for treatment approval varies from about $30,000 to $75,000 per year of life saved (or QALY, quality-adjusted years of life saved). But many treatments that are more expensive are still used and approved. Treatment for hypercholesterolemia with statin drugs (like Lipitor), and mammography in women aged forty to fifty are two examples of "expensive" tests and treatments, since they cost more than $75,000 per year of life saved. But they are still considered standard of care for patients. And while the cost of any treatment is easy to determine, clinical scientists often do not have survival data on many treatments; therefore, their cost/benefit ratio is still unknown.

## Complementary and Alternative Medicine

The Internet, newspapers, and all media are filled with reports about and advertisements for alternative treatments that their manufacturers want you to buy. Inevitably, each report or ad is accompanied by patient testimonials telling how well the product works. But are the testimonials true?

Alternative therapy is unproven treatment given in place of standard treatments. Complementary therapy is unproven treatment that is given together with standard therapy. Almost no alternative or complementary therapies have had clinical trials demonstrating effectiveness that have been published in peer-reviewed journals. (These are journals that won't publish the trials unless they've been reviewed by specialists to verify that the results were proven.) Because of the broad public interest in these usually nutritional- or vitamin-based approaches to health care, the National Institutes of Health is doing research on many of these therapies. Most have shown no effectiveness.

But how can you know what is "snake oil" and what has real promise? Do some research on the Internet, and then check with your doctor or specialist. Here are some high-profile alternative or complementary treatments—and what we know about their effectiveness:

- We used to hear that laetrile and vitamin C helped fight cancer. Large national trials showed that neither works. You shouldn't consider them.
- We had heard that the spice turmeric could help fight cancer. Now we know that an active ingredient of turmeric, curcumin, actually can effectively kill cancer cells in the test tube, and it is now in clinical trials. So you might try turmeric, with your doctor's advice.
- Asian people have long claimed that green tea is an anticancer agent. Now recent studies have shown that an active component of green tea called EGCG (epigallocatechin gallate) kills cancer cells in the lab. You might consider using green tea, if your doctor agrees.
- Some women have claimed that black cohosh reduced their hot flashes, but large clinical trials showed that the plant was no more effective than sugar pills in easing that menopause symptom. Some antidepressants did work better, however, so consider the medicines, not the cohosh.

Here's the bottom line with alternative or complementary treatments: always check with your doctor, preferably a specialist. If she cannot answer your questions or recommend other, more effective medicines and nutrients, ask about a second opinion.

### Tips

- If you're considering an alternative or complementary treatment, first ask your physician a few questions: "Is there more benefit or more risk in this treatment for me? Is there a practice guideline that you are following? If you were me, what would you do?" Your doctor's answers will help you make an informed decision about whether that treatment is worth using and worth a fight to obtain authorization.

- Consider a second opinion from another specialist more familiar with the treatment under consideration. This may convince you of the usefulness of the treatment—or its questionable nature—and help you decide whether to pursue it. The report from such a consultation can also support your appeal if your insurance company initially denied the treatment.
- Disease support groups can offer recommendations about different treatments. With their input, you can better understand whether your physician said "there's no proof" to support certain treatments simply because the results of clinical trials are unclear, or because insurance restrictions or other extraneous factors are impeding your access to appropriate or promising treatments.
- Ask the physician, "What evidence is there to support the use of the treatment or show that it doesn't work, and what have been the results in other treatment centers, universities, or international trials?" These questions will reveal your doctor's knowledge of a particular treatment and the reasons why he did not recommend it.
- Ask, "Is this treatment actually not helpful, or is it just too expensive to be authorized?" If cost is the issue, keep in mind that pharmaceutical companies occasionally will supply a new drug to a doctor for free through what is called a "compassionate use" program, or they can help you and your doctor fight for authorization.
- Sometimes the cost of a treatment is so low that patients just pay for it themselves. If you end up doing this, still appeal the lack of payment to your insurance company or the state board of insurance, because many insurance companies will ultimately pay for previously denied treatments.

## Contemporary Medicine and Medical Proof

As medicine becomes more expensive, health-care reforms are continuously pushing back on the overuse of unproven therapies. Insurers typically say that an unproven treatment is "experimental" and therefore not covered by their plan. Or they will conclude that although a certain treatment is effective, a cheaper method works just as well and must be tried first. These sorts of policies are ubiquitous within the insurance industry, so if you've had an illness, you probably have experienced them.

As trials increasingly measure the cost-benefit ratio and cost per QALY, insurance companies will increasingly deny coverage for possibly breakthrough treatments. (A recent example is the drug bevacizumab for treatment of breast cancers.)

If you experience such denials, get a second opinion from a specialist—usually someone affiliated with a university. Often his or her letter of support for a treatment can persuade your insurance company to reverse its decision. It's also possible that the second opinion may convince you that the new, expensive medicine you wanted really *won't* help you, so you can feel more confident about the older, less expensive therapy. Either way, you win.

# Chapter 17

# The Cutting Edge: Clinical Trials

As a science, medicine is not perfect. Doctors are controlling and curing many diseases with more success than ever before. But we still face challenges to successfully treat many other diseases, such as lung cancer, pancreatic cancer, stroke, emphysema, cirrhosis, macular degeneration, deafness, spinal injury, and neurologic diseases such as Alzheimer's. And although we have developed good treatments for common diseases like diabetes, coronary artery disease, colitis, kidney failure, arthritis, and muscular dystrophy, we have not yet discovered their cures.

Because of these imperfect results, medicine is always trying to improve its treatments and outcomes. As far back as the sixteenth century, physicians published books of their successful outcomes. For example, the favorable results of patient treatments administered by Shakespeare's father-in-law, John Hall, were published just after his death as a guide for other doctors.

Medical journals were regularly published in the 1800s, when physicians would share their personal experiences regarding individual patients and promising new treatments (often herbs, medicines, or improved surgical techniques). These collections of anecdotal results were replaced during the early and middle 1900s by publications documenting the results of formal, well-designed clinical trials.

Clinical trials can be very helpful to individual patients. Years ago my patient Doug had developed Kaposi's sarcoma, a cancer of his skin, leg, and lungs related to his AIDS. Despite his treatment with all the available chemotherapy known to be useful, the ugly brown spots and pain continued to progress, so I told Doug about a new drug delivered by microscopic fat bubbles (liposomes); it had just been approved for initial clinical trials. After hearing and reading about the risks and benefits of the treatment, Doug agreed to participate in the clinical trial and signed all the forms allowing us to proceed. A few weeks later, when Doug returned for evaluation, he was thrilled with the results. "I can't believe how well this new drug is working," he told me. "Look at these nodules on my face—they're completely flat and have started to fade. I'm off all the pain medicine now. My leg is nearly back to normal size, and I don't have to use those awful elastic wraps anymore." Doug's remission in his cancer lasted twelve months on the clinical trial. Because of his results and those of a hundred other patients on that clinical trial, the drug was approved by the FDA and became available to patients throughout the country.

## What are Clinical Trials?

A clinical trial is a study of a new treatment, procedure, or diagnostic test in a set number of patients (the sample population). The trial assesses the usefulness (benefit) and/or the side effects (risk) of the intervention. If the test involves a small number of patients (fewer than twenty), the results must be cautiously interpreted because so few patient experiences were observed. If the study is large (hundreds to thousands of patients), its conclusions are more likely to be accurate, because there is much less chance of misinterpreting the results.

In "nonrandomized" clinical trials, every patient gets the same treatment. In larger "randomized" trials, some patients get one treatment and some get another; they are placed at random (by chance) into one of two treatments, called "arm one" and "arm two." (There may be more than two treatments or "arms," depending on the clinical study.) When the trial is finished, the results of each arm are compared to those of the other(s) to see which one worked best.

In randomized trials, one treatment is the "control arm"—the standard treatment physicians already use. The other treatments are the "test" or "experimental" arms—the new treatments that are being investigated to see if they are better or worse than the control treatment. If you participate in a randomized clinical trial, here is your dilemma: you don't get to choose whether you'll receive the new treatment, because your assignment to a control arm or to the new test arm is computerized, made by chance only. So should you participate or not? I'll give you my recommendations in a few more paragraphs, but first let's find out a little more about clinical trials.

## Regulation of Clinical Trials

In the past, clinical trials were conducted solely at universities and large research centers. Today, however, they are conducted in almost every community, including many hospitals and physicians' offices as well as universities, research centers, and independent institutes. In fact, your own doctor may be participating in clinical trials. (If she is, that's a good sign she practices quality medicine, as participation in clinical trials helps keep doctors current. So ask your doctor if clinical trials are available at her practice.)

Clinical trials came under government regulation after World War II, when it was revealed that concentration camp prisoners were subjected to cruel medical experimentation by government-employed doctors, resulting in suffering, mutilation, and often death. The Nuremberg Code of Medical Ethics formed the basis for subsequent clinical trial law and has been implemented in most countries, including the United States. Clinical trials now are strictly regulated based on national and international standards. American clinical trials designed to evaluate new drugs or devices are overseen by the FDA as well as the federal Office for Human Research Protection (OHRP).

Today, if you are considering participating in a clinical trial, all the following conditions must have been met before the new treatment can begin:

- The clinical trial must have been approved by an investigational review board (IRB), which considers the scientific basis for the trial and its potential risks and benefits, and which ensures that all the paperwork you will sign is understandable and clearly informs you of the potential risks and benefits.

- You must meet all the patient eligibility criteria for entering the study.
- You must have reviewed the information about the study, which is described in the informed consent document outlining the potential risks and benefits, and you must have given your written consent to participate.

To ensure the safety of participants, each trial is continuously monitored by the local investigational review board or, in some cases, a national board. Some trials are also periodically reviewed (audited) by the federal government. If a trial fails to pass such an audit, all clinical research at that center must stop. Therefore doctors and the university or research center are under pressure to conduct all trials effectively, honestly, and comprehensively to comply with all the procedures and steps defined in the trial.

## Benefits and Cautions about Clinical Trials

With all the cumbersome machinery regulating clinical trials, why should you consider participating in one? Well, it can offer you the chance for better results than you'd get with standard care, and it helps society by giving doctors the ability to test new types of treatments. And a clinical trial is usually the only way a patient can access one of the thousands of new drugs being tested for life-threatening illnesses.

Be aware of a cautionary note, however: some trials have had unacceptably bad side effects, like the birth defects produced by the medication thalidomide, or the increased risk of heart attack with some newer anti-arthritis drugs. So before entering a clinical trial, make sure you read and understand all the information contained in the informed consent document. Ask questions and get clear answers from the doctors, nurses, or clinical trial monitors who review the informed consent document with you.

It should take you much longer to consider a clinical trial than a standard treatment. Allow yourself enough time to weigh all the risks and benefits; you might want to take the consent documents home to read very carefully, rather than rushing a decision in the doctor's office. Look up the clinical trial online by typing "patient experience with drug XXX" in a search engine. You can often find comments posted by patients who have participated in the same or similar trials. Their input can help you decide if a certain trial is for you.

Has your physician or the clinical trials nurse (or monitor) spent adequate time discussing these treatments with you? Is your physician participating in clinical trials? If you were offered the opportunity to participate in a clinical trial, would the unknown potential side effects worry you, or would the risk be worth whatever benefits you might gain from the investigational treatment?

## When to Consider Participating in a Clinical Trial

For most patients, the decision to participate in a clinical trial depends on their answers to some critical questions:

- How severe is your illness?
- How frightened are you about your prognosis?
- How severe are your symptoms?
- How badly does the disease affect your life?
- How much risk do you want to take to try to get better?
- How much do you trust the doctor proposing the clinical trial?
- Are there any standard treatments available for your illness?
- How does the clinical trial treatment compare to the standard alternative, if there is one?

If you want better-than-usual results, you should consider a clinical trial. However, if you do not want to risk the possibility of getting worse results or more toxicity than you would from usual or standard treatments, you should probably opt out of the clinical trial and look for the best standard care instead.

What is the right path to take? If you are facing a serious condition or life-threatening disease, I recommend that you ask your doctor about any clinical trials that are available to you. But don't stop there—do your own research to learn what is going on in research trials.

## Where to Find a Clinical Trial

First, ask your own doctor if a clinical trial is available for your illness. Physicians who specialize in a disease usually know what trials are available for it, but if your doctor is unfamiliar with what is available for you, ask for a referral to a center studying your type of disease. Often this is a large community hospital or university center, so you may have to travel a bit to get there, but invariably it is worth the effort.

Once you have been given information about a clinical trial, you must decide whether you are interested in participating. If you are having a hard time deciding, ask the physician conducting the trial, "If this were you, what would you do? Would you take the regular therapy, or would you participate in this clinical trial?" Almost every honest investigator will answer this question, so beware of a doctor who won't.

If you are still undecided, consider getting a second opinion about the clinical trial from a physician who is not involved in it but who is still very knowledgeable about the nature of the trial. You can sometimes get a different perspective about the proposed tests or treatments from someone outside the medical center hosting the trial. A specialist from another large center or university can help you decide, even if it means a trip to another city.

## If Your Doctor Won't Refer You to a Clinical Trial

This situation is not uncommon—you are interested in learning about clinical trials, but your doctor will not refer you to one or doesn't know anyone conducting clinical trials that might be appropriate for you. What should you do next?

Fortunately, there are national lists of all trials available for all diseases (except for the occasional isolated trial in a smaller institution). You can find these lists, and the contact information you'll need to find out if you're eligible to participate, on the Internet at CenterWatch.com. Look under "Find Clinical Trials," "Search Clinical Trials," and "Overview of Clinical Trials." I also recommend calling other medical centers in your community or a local university hospital (ask for the department that cares for your illness) to inquire if trials are available. Usually there is a trial coordinator who can discuss this with you.

Once you've found a clinical trial, determine if you are eligible to participate in it. Often the entry criteria for a trial are very strict, and doctors who violate these rules of entry for any patient risk losing their ability to participate in trials again. If you are interested in a trial but are deemed ineligible, ask the physician if you might be eligible for a trial of the same treatment at another hospital or medical center. Or go online and search "clinical trials for treatment XXX."

## Other Sources of Information on Clinical Trials

Many organizations and agencies have websites offering important information on clinical trials, including how to participate and potential risks. Some of these Internet resources can help you or your family to locate a clinical trial and decide whether to participate in it. They also can give you more information that can stimulate questions for you to ask the doctor. Consider visiting these websites:

- National Institutes of Health: ClinicalTrials.gov
- The Center for Information and Study on Clinical Research Participation: CISCRP.org
- The National Clinical Trials Listing Service: CenterWatch.com
- National Cancer Institute: Cancer.gov
- National Coalition for Cancer Survivorship: CancerAdvocacy.org

## Information about the Trial

Once you have decided to consider a clinical trial, there are questions you should ask the doctor conducting the research or the research coordinator (sometimes called a "trial monitor"):

**Is the physician disclosing all his reasons for suggesting a new clinical trial, or does he have a conflict of interest?** Many physicians or centers are paid to enroll patients into a clinical trial—as much as $2,000 to $15,000 per patient. While this is completely legal and generally necessary because of the time and effort needed to conduct the trial, some physicians' income or employment is largely dependent upon putting a certain number of patients on clinical trials. So is this clinical trial really in your best interest, or is it being suggested to you because the physician wants to protect his job or increase his income? Many times, a physician owns stock in the company that is producing the new treatment, or he may even have developed the treatment personally. Has the physician disclosed all this to you or reassured you that there is no conflict of interest? Keep in mind that even if the physician does have a conflict of interest, the clinical trial might still be the best possible treatment for you. You should just know all the facts before you decide. You might delicately ask, "I know it takes a lot of effort to do a study like this … Do you get paid for putting me on it?" or, "You are at the cutting edge of this research. Have you developed this study yourself, and do you have stock in or own a part of the company sponsoring the study?" If the answer is yes, your follow-up question might be, "In the interest of disclosure, which I know you have to follow, how much?"

**Can you be assured you'll actually get the new, experimental treatment?** In many trials, the new treatment is compared to a placebo, so participants might be selected by chance to receive nothing at all. Some new treatments are in such short supply that participants are accepted by lottery—as happened with the multiple sclerosis treatment interferon, whose limited availability required that only a few patients per month be entered in the trial.

**Will you have to pay anything for the experimental treatment?** If so, how much—and can you afford it? Is your physician actually approved to give the experimental treatment to you? Will you have to undergo additional tests, X-rays, or biopsies in addition to what would be considered standard therapy, and if so, who will pay for them?

**Has an investigational review board reviewed the trial?** Can you get a copy of the approval? Is the research program approved by the FDA?

**Will your health insurance approve your participation in this trial?** If so, you can probably receive the investigational treatment (which might be free and not billed to the insurance) and all the tests required (which often are billed to insurance), plus the costs of supportive care if you develop a complication. If not, your insurance company likely will refuse to pay for your care while you are on the clinical trial. The Patient Protection and Affordable Care Act requires most private insurance plans to cover the usual care costs while patients are on many clinical trials, and Medicare has a similar provision. To be certain if your care will be covered by your insurance, ask the physician and also your insurance company.

**Has the physician proposing the clinical trial also disclosed all the standard options to you?** This is required by international standards and federal law. In some centers that specialize in investigational treatments, you may remain under the care of a doctor at the center only if you participate in a clinical trial—which can put pressure on you to accept the trial. Know in advance whether the doctor will still take care of you or refer you elsewhere if you decline to participate in a trial and opt for standard therapy.

### Tips

- If you are concerned about the limited effectiveness of a standard treatment program, always ask about clinical trials. If your physician does not know about relevant clinical trials, ask to be referred for a second opinion to another center where you can discuss them.
- When you see a physician who is offering a clinical trial, always ask for time to read the informed consent document completely, and ask the physician to explain any words that you do not understand. If you have persistent questions, write them down and ask the investigator of the trial. If the physician and the physician's staff still do not adequately explain them to you, be wary of participating in that clinical trial.

## My Personal Advice about Participating

- If I just had a mild illness with no long-term disability or reduced quality of life, I would be reluctant to enter a clinical trial.
- If I had a serious illness, I would always ask about clinical trials.
- If a standard treatment existed and the trial compared that standard therapy with a new and promising treatment, I would carefully evaluate the new treatment and get a second opinion about participating.
- If a standard treatment existed but the trial compared a new investigational treatment to no treatment at all (or a placebo, and you must be told if a placebo is being used), I would not participate unless I could *later* get the new treatment after the placebo and *later* also get the standard treatment. In other words, don't burn your bridges: always keep your options open to get the standard treatments and, if possible, the investigational treatment as well.
- If a standard treatment existed but the trial involved just a new, experimental treatment (not a randomized trial, but one with only one treatment arm, the experimental treatment), I would consider it, but I would also get a second opinion about the new treatment. Then I would ask, "After the experimental treatment, can I still get the standard treatment?"
- If I had a serious illness for which there was no standard treatment, or for which I had already been through all the standard treatments, I would always seek out a clinical trial. If my doctor didn't know of one, I would get a second opinion from another specialist who had such trials available, even if I had to travel to a university in another city.

I strongly encourage my patients to consider clinical trials when standard therapy is less than optimal. Clinical trials are the superhighway to improving medical care for ourselves, our families, and our children. Without clinical trials and patients willing to participate in them, medicine would not be able to make the progress that leads to longer and happier lives.

## Today's Medicine and Clinical Trials

Several new trends in clinical trials are emerging as a result of health-care reform. The first is insurance companies' increased willingness to allow you to enter clinical trials. As long as the trial pays for much of your care, any new procedures or drugs, and any extra tests over and above standard-care tests, insurance will probably authorize the clinical care costs of such investigational study programs. Medicare is committed to this process, but only for certain trials. Find out in advance what costs will be paid for by your insurance plan by asking both your insurance company and the physician offering the trial. Being forewarned avoids frustration and expense later.

Since care through university or tertiary-care specialty hospitals is often more expensive than care by a doctor in your health plan, some insurance programs (particularly HMOs and heavily managed plans) may be reluctant to authorize second opinions obtained at such hospitals. If you want to get to them, you may have to appeal a denial with your insurance plan, or even go to the state insurance commissioner's office to help you get permission and payment for the second opinion.

Keep in mind, also, that with the increased use of nurse practitioners and physicians' assistants, you may be treated by health-care professionals who are not knowledgeable about clinical trials. To make sure you're getting the best information, ask them to check with the doctor about clinical trials for you, or speak to the doctor yourself.

# Chapter 18

# How to Get More and Better Care in a Hospital

Although much of this book has dealt with interactions between you and your physician, medical care for very serious illnesses and operations typically occurs in hospitals. While most hospitals give good care, no hospital is free from error, and no hospital gives perfect care to every patient. Why? As with doctors' offices, hospitals are facing intense pressures on several levels. The major problem is financial, since many hospitals are facing budget deficits due to reduced payments from insurance companies and Medicare and Medicaid. Such hospitals often cut their payroll costs by employing fewer nurses to care for patients. With so many patients and the increasing seriousness of their illnesses, hospital employees suffer from stress and work overload. The busier nurses are, the harder it is to get their attention to take care of your problems and administer your medicine on time.

Furthermore, as hospitals attempt to improve their quality of care, they have increased their requirements for nurses to document patient conditions and treatments—record keeping that further reduces the time they spend with you. And as hospitals seek to raise the quality of the nursing staff by requiring more in-service training, fewer nurses are left at the bedside to care for you. On top of that, shortages of available nurses and technicians in the job market also promote understaffing. Fewer staff and less hands-on care lead to poor medical outcomes, errors in care, and unhappy patients and families.

After developing pneumonia, my patient Nancy—a prominent businesswoman and active mother—was admitted to the hospital for intravenous antibiotics. When I saw Nancy the next day, she was in tears. "They just wouldn't come," she said. "I just called and called—I needed a urinal—and all they said was that the nurses were busy and they'd get to me when they could. And they never came, and here I am, lying in a mess. I'm so mad. This has never happened to me before—at least, not since I was four!" Furious, I went to the nursing supervisor to complain. The supervisor explained, "You know we've been having this staffing problem. We have some registry nurses who are not our regular staff, and sometimes they don't come when they should. I'll check into it, and it won't happen again." But it has happened, again and again, despite no one—not the patients, their families, or the nurses, supervisors, or doctors—wanting it to.

Another patient, Patty, had been admitted to the hospital for a pleural effusion, or fluid around her lung. After a tube was inserted to drain the fluid, I thought I'd find her much more comfortable and smiling. But when I visited her several days later, she said, "Doctor Presant, why do you have me in this awful hospital? The aides came to help me go to the toilet, but that was four days ago! Yesterday, no nurse came, and they didn't seem to even know I was here. My husband, Bob, has become my chief potty emptier, and after he took care of me, he had to get up to take my roommate to the toilet, since no one came to help her after she pushed the call button. Last night, I finally saw a nurse. She came in and woke me up at midnight to say hello and ask if I needed something." After hearing Patty's complaints, I called the president of the hospital and then the vice president of nursing and patient care. Once the chief administrators heard about her poor care, Patty started getting more attention. After her breathing normalized and the chest catheter was removed, Patty and Bob even brought thank-you candy for the nurses who were finally showing her the compassion and attention she should have been receiving all along.

What can you expect to experience in the hospital nowadays? In general, you will probably get less attention by nurses and possibly more mistakes in your care. A study by the Institute of Medicine, a nonprofit group of prestigious physicians, found that the error rate in medicine is high, resulting in forty-four thousand to ninety-eight thousand hospital deaths per year. These errors are commonly due to miscommunication or poor compliance with hospital rules. It stands to reason that if hospital staff have less time to double-check orders or patient care, mistakes can be made. According to one report, 7 percent of hospitalized patients suffer from an adverse drug reaction, and many of these reactions are preventable.

Many errors in medication dosing have resulted in patient deaths, and administering the wrong medication has resulted in severe patient suffering. When there are fewer pharmacists and nurses, patient care becomes rushed. You could be one of these casualties of the hospital system if the nurses, doctor, and staff involved in your care are not cautious.

Almost every hospital in America conducts patient satisfaction surveys, and many will make the results available if you go to the hospital administration or nursing director's offices and ask for them. Hospitals commonly use the Press-Ganey study results, since a poor score motivates administrators to make changes. Good scores on these patient surveys are closely associated both with better patient outcomes (fewer medication errors, shorter hospital stays) and with more economic stability in the hospital (which usually means better staffing and therefore more attention to patients). If the scores seem poor to you, ask to speak to the head of nursing administration to say that you expect truly excellent care—better than you see in the survey results.

The best predictor of patient satisfaction is prompt and complete attention to any complaint or question. If you receive slow attention or a delayed response from the nursing staff, you or your family should complain aggressively all the way up the chain of command. Start with the nurses, but continue on, as necessary, to the nursing supervisor, the chief nursing administrator, the president or CEO, and the chairman of the board. On the other hand, if you receive good, timely care, commend the staff members who helped you get good care.

Reviewing your hospital records for accuracy can both reassure you that the quality of your care has been good, and help identify possible problems. Inaccuracies can be corrected, and omissions can be filled in. These are important documents that should be correct and later added to your personal medical record (see appendix 1).

The hospital staff's attention to and attitude about their patients' problems are evident in the types of observations and notes they make in their records, so reading those records can be your special quality control check to ensure you've received high-quality care. When one of my patients collected her records from a prominent hospital to which she had been referred, she was astonished to find that a hospital employee had forged her signature on a consent form for a liver biopsy. She never returned to that hospital. If that can happen at one of the nation's finest hospitals, it can happen in a hospital you might use. So be aware, ask for copies of records, and read them carefully.

Strategic scheduling of medical procedures and testing is important for obtaining the best results. One of my patients got a mammogram on a Friday and was told by the technician that there was something suspicious, but no physician was available to review the result until Monday (doctors frequently do not work weekends except in emergencies). She was a nervous wreck for days until the abnormality was found to be just a normal variant. The lesson: never have an elective nonemergency test or procedure or operation on a Friday or around the time of a holiday weekend. Since staffing is less complete (nurses and staff take off extra time around holidays too), attention to problems can be deficient and errors may occur.

Ask your doctor to recommend the best time for you to get a particular treatment. Hospital and/or office staff also can advise you whether staffing may be spotty during the times you are considering for surgery or treatments. Knowing the doctor's vacation schedule helps you determine your best timing for medical care, which can assure you the best follow-up results and the fastest recovery from any operation.

## Hospital Errors in Diagnosis

The most important aspect of your health care is getting the right diagnosis. Unfortunately, some diagnoses are wrong and therefore the wrong treatments are given. When you are in the hospital, a diagnosis is usually made based on a test, X-ray, biopsy, or surgery. Most doctors make one hundred to one thousand decisions per day, and errors occur.

Sometimes it's not your attending doctor (the one who admitted you and whose name is on your chart), or even one of your consulting specialist physicians, who makes the mistake. The radiologist interpreting your X-rays can miss an important finding; I've read that 30 percent of radiologist opinions are incorrect. But in my experience, it's more like 2 or 3 percent, since I usually use hospitals with several radiologists who check difficult findings with each other. So check with your doctor to see whether you will use a radiology group whose doctors help each other diagnose challenging cases.

The pathologist, another doctor you never see, can make a mistake in interpreting a biopsy. After you have a biopsy or operation, the tissue from the biopsy is sent to the pathologist, who examines it under a microscope to be certain of the diagnosis. An often-quoted statistic is that more than 20 percent of autopsies show diseases that were not diagnosed by the patients' physicians.

How can you protect yourself against an incorrect or missed diagnosis and wrong treatments? When a doctor tells you what is wrong with you, ask the following important questions:

- How certain are you of the diagnosis?
- Could there be an error in the diagnosis?
- If my diagnosis is based on a biopsy or an X-ray, can you have another pathologist or radiologist review it, or could you send it to an outside expert for confirmation?

Within any hospital, there is almost always more than one radiologist and pathologist from whom a second opinion is immediately available. Beyond that, you can easily arrange through your doctor to get the critical test or biopsy reviewed by an outside physician expert—you just have to ask. Since a correct diagnosis is crucial to your care, don't hesitate to ask for your doctor's help as soon as possible. You or your family may have to take the X-ray films or the actual pathology slides to another hospital yourselves in order to get the outside opinion, but usually this is faster than relying on the first hospital to send out your biopsy slides or X-rays via mail.

If you are told that your test indicates you need an operation, consider getting a second surgical consultation to be certain that the surgery is needed and that the right surgery is being planned by the right surgeon. The second-opinion doctor should have his own pathologist or radiologist confirm the findings upon which your diagnosis depends.

Also, if you are told you have a life-threatening disease, get a second opinion to be certain of the diagnosis.

## Patient Advocates

When you are in the hospital as an inpatient, you will be very vulnerable. If you are very ill, or if you are reluctant to ask any questions yourself (as many patients are), or if you are sleepy or even confused from medication, it may help to have a family member or friend—an "advocate"—ask questions on your behalf to your physician or nurses.

*If you do not have a patient advocate staying with you or visiting you daily to help you make decisions and to watch over you, then it is most important that you act as your own advocate. Your life could depend on it.*

What is a "patient advocate," and can having another person with you always help you get better care? A patient advocate is someone you designate to be with you—typically in the hospital, but also in the doctor's office, if you desire. This person helps you understand what the doctors and nurses are telling you, helps you ask questions, and watches out for you. The advocate checks your medicines and tests and makes your complaints known to your nurse or doctor. Some people recommend choosing an advocate who is familiar with the medical system and can spend a lot of time with you. Although having an advocate with some medical training or familiarity is not fundamentally important (just a little helpful), having an advocate who really cares about you and will ask important questions is an absolute necessity.

Advocates have been around for a long time … they just weren't called "advocates." When you were a child, your parent who took you to the doctor's office was your advocate. And even when you get sick as an adult, you may ask a parent, child, sibling, spouse, or close friend to be at the doctor's office with you to help you listen and understand. But now, with doctors' offices and hospitals rushing their patient care, having a buddy to help you is more important than ever. It doesn't need to be the same person all the time, but the advocate needs to be someone whom you can trust completely with your most private information, someone to whom you can always talk, and someone with enough emotional strength not to be overwhelmed by your problems.

To work well with your advocate, you must be honest with her so she realizes not only how much she can help, but also how much responsibility may be required of her. It can take time, effort, and commitment to be an effective advocate. That said, spouses and close family rarely object to shouldering that burden.

Remember how, in prior chapters, I stressed the importance of bringing a close family member or friend with you to the doctor? Well, that's even more important in the hospital. While you're an inpatient, ask your doctor if your family or friend can sleep over with you in your room, since many patients' needs arise at night. The doctor can write an order permitting this in most instances, though usually not in the intensive care unit (ICU). Make sure all the doctors and nurses know whom you have selected to help you (give them a list of all the names if there are several people), and let them know that they have your permission to discuss your situation with your advocate at any time. Be sure that your advocate's phone numbers— as well as those of any important family members—are on your chart both in the hospital and in your doctors' offices.

Your hospital roommate—that is, the patient in the other bed—will not make a good advocate. He or she may be too ill to help or to make good judgments. Even if a roommate has helped you once by calling a nurse for you, that person may not be able to make the call the next time.

To help you specify the role you want your advocate to play and to help him understand what he needs to do, the following list may be helpful. Go over it with him to make sure he knows all the ways he can help you.

## The Advocate's Role in the Hospital

### Patient Protection

- Call the nurse and doctor for the patient.
- Know the names of the nurses, aides, and pharmacist, and have the phone number of the nurse (cell phone) or nurse's station. Know which shifts they work. Call them by name.
- Know the name of and talk to the nursing supervisor. Complain when you're getting bad care, and praise the nurses when they give you great care.

- If there are problems in your care, complain directly to the nursing supervisor, director of nursing, CEO, or hospital board chairman.
- Request medications as needed for pain, anxiety, diarrhea, nausea, heartburn, etc.
- Ask for a pharmacist to review all medications.
- Keep track of all tests and their results.
- Keep a list of questions for the nurses or doctors (and write down their answers).
- Ask questions on behalf of the patient.
- Check all medications given.
- Check that any blood product transfusion is really intended for you and not someone else.
- Check patient ID before the patient is taken for procedures.
- Be certain each nurse, doctor, orderly, visitor, and therapist washes his or her hands before touching the patient.
- Be certain all meals and drinks are on the prescribed diet.
- Check on test results if they have not been reported.
- Check when medications and treatments are due, keep a schedule, and call if they are not on time.
- Call the doctor about treatment questions.

**Patient Advice**
- Provide encouragement to the patient.
- Get visitors in and out on time.
- Convey any information the patient wants to tell family and friends.
- Discuss problems with the patient.
- Provide activities, books, magazines, music, and/or videos to keep the patient's mind active and avoid depression.
- Help with physical therapy and exercise (as consistent with doctors' orders).
- Help the patient get second opinions if necessary.
- Provide emotional support before procedures (hold hands).
- Be present when the procedures are completed and the patient returns to bed.
- Arrange for coverage if the advocate needs to be absent.

- Keep names posted of doctors, nurses, aids, therapists, case manager, discharge planner, social services contact, and pharmacist.
- Keep a calendar posted.
- Post cards, pictures, and arrange flowers for a supportive environment.
- Get hospital bills before discharge and review them with the patient.
- Arrange for the pharmacist to visit and go over patient medications before discharge.
- Decide if more supportive help is needed.
- Help the patient to get information from the Internet, if needed.
- Assist with social services help and discharge planning.
- Keep copies of medical records and test results.

**Patient Comfort**
- Get water, drinks, and snacks.
- Help with meals.
- Bring in outside food, if approved by doctor.
- Help with bed position, pillows, gown, bedpan, baths, and walking.
- Answer the phone and take messages.
- Make phone calls to family, friends, or work, at the direction of the patient.
- Keep track of patient's clothes and protect any valuables.

## How Long Should Your Hospitalization Last?

Generally, patients get well in hospitals … but not always. Some patients actually get sicker in hospitals. So how long should you stay?

First, if you can avoid being in the hospital, do. Try to remain an outpatient. Even if you need a lot of tests, which can be inconvenient as an outpatient because you need to go back and forth for all the test appointments, try to avoid being hospitalized. Serious errors occur in hospitals, and very serious infections can be acquired from other patients.

But if you don't have a choice because you are severely ill or need surgery, be certain your doctor knows you want to stay long enough to have your illness diagnosed or your condition improve, so that you will not get sicker right after discharge and require readmission. If you need surgery, a biopsy, or even a second opinion during your hospital stay, tell your doctor that you want it done as soon as possible.

That said, you should also tell your doctors that you do not want to remain in the hospital longer than necessary, since you could get complications. The frequency of acquiring a life-threatening antibiotic-resistant infection increases by 1 percent with each day of hospital stay. To shorten your stay, be sure your doctor has ordered a dietician evaluation and physical therapy, if necessary, to get you back on your feet and keep you strong for home, and as many specialists as necessary to make your diagnosis and therapy more efficient. If you are weak or wobbly when you walk, be sure that a physical therapist or nurse helps you out of bed, and that nurses and aides keep your bed rails up. If your roommate has an infection, ask to be transferred to another room so you do not catch it. And don't let sick relatives or friends visit you and share their infections with you.

## Pathways to Better Hospital Care

When you go to the hospital, bring a list of all your medications, including doses, and a copy of your personal medical record, and show it to the nurse who admits you to the hospital floor. (Don't give it to the nurse, though; always keep it by your bedside, since these records can get lost at the nursing station.) If the nurse wants to keep it with your inpatient chart, ask which records they need and then have your advocate or family member make a copy, while you keep the original. Point out your specific medical-care needs, your allergies, and the list of all your conditions and illnesses.

Check your medications each time you receive them. Show your wristband identification to the nurse giving you the medicine to be certain it is your own medication. Ask which medications you're being given, and why. If you don't recognize a new medicine, ask the nurse to identify it so you can check the pills each time you get them. If you have any questions about your medicines, ask to speak to the hospital pharmacist; there is usually one assigned to each patient unit in the hospital, and they like talking to patients and answering questions.

If you are going to be given intravenous fluid or a blood transfusion, check that your name is actually on the bag by having the nurse show it to you. If you are receiving blood, be certain it is the correct blood type.

If you are having an operation on one arm or leg or on one side of your body, put a little sign on your body saying "This one" and a sign on the other side saying "Not this one." Unfortunately, there have been instances of surgeons operating on the wrong side.

Be certain everyone who is examining you (including your doctor, nurse, nurse's aide, and radiologist) washes his or her hands before touching you.

Know how to call the nurse from your hospital bed, and have a bell or whistle by your bed in the event that your call button is not working. Since even those measures sometimes fail to bring a nurse, keep a mobile phone nearby so you can call your family, your doctor, and the nursing unit responsible for your care.

In order to reemphasize this important point, I am repeating it here. **Always have the people caring for you wash their hands with soap and water or use an antimicrobial gel before touching you.** The easiest way to prevent serious infections is to avoid exposure, and many hospital personnel carry germs from one patient to another. In an emergency room, nearly every employee and doctor can transmit antibiotic-resistant germs, so be certain they wash thoroughly or use gloves before examining or treating you.

Your doctors should know what tests have been done prior to your hospital stay so that retesting is avoided. Even so, it's a good idea to bring a copy of your personal medical record to the hospital to remind them. (Leave the original at home so it doesn't get lost.) Ask your nurses if anything can be done to speed up your hospitalization. And ask to speak to a discharge planner early during your stay so that you can begin anticipating and finding solutions to your home needs. This will help prevent a delay in discharge.

If you've had surgery, make sure that your bandages (dressings) are changed often during your hospital stay to avoid wound infections or poor healing. (Your surgeon can tell you on your first post-operative day how often the dressings need to be changed, and then you can remind the nurses if they have not been changed.) If you are in a teaching hospital, make certain that your attending, board-certified doctor evaluates you every day and that your questions are answered daily by your doctor—not an intern, resident, fellow, or medical student.

If you have more than one doctor looking in on you—which is nearly universal in the hospital, with so many consultants needed to address complicated illnesses—ask each doctor every day for the results of your recent tests. Ask them if they have personally seen those test results and discussed them with the other doctors and especially your attending physician, so that your care is coordinated and efficient. Keep a pad by your bedside to write down all your questions and concerns so you don't forget.

Demand excellent care. If you have a problem with your care, complain immediately to your physician and your nursing supervisor. Then write letters to the president and the chairman of the board of the hospital, and ask to discuss the problems with them or their representative. Similarly, if you are getting good care, write letters to the president and the chairman of the board and thank them for it. Let the nurses and the nursing supervisors know how happy you have been with the care they provided. Consider bringing in a small gift or pizza or candy for the nurses, aides, and clerks who have participated in your care, just as you would for a friend who has done you a favor.

If you need to use the emergency room, tell the emergency-room receptionist about any life-threatening symptoms: chest pain, arm pain, palpitations, bleeding, fainting, paralysis, or seizure. *Do not minimize any of your symptoms; more serious symptoms are always taken care of more quickly.* If you are having chest pains or fear you are having heart-related symptoms, call an ambulance to take you to the hospital. *Paramedic arrivals are always evaluated more quickly.* Be certain the emergency-room personnel know the names of your primary doctor and your consultants; if the ER calls them upon your arrival, it will speed up your care.

When you're discharged from the hospital, ask your nurse to review all your instructions with you. And although you'll probably want to get out of there as quickly as possible, to be thorough you should have a checklist of discharge activities that must take place prior to your exit:

1. Have a follow-up appointment set up with each of your doctors. Make sure you have an address, phone, fax, and e-mail for each.

2. Have all your prescriptions (checked to ensure they are the same dose you have been receiving in the hospital), preferably with instructions from both the nurse and the hospital pharmacist. These instructions should include information about the risks or benefits of any new medication you will begin taking at home. If you have any questions about why you have to take them or how to take them, ask to speak to the pharmacist directly.

3. Get written instructions regarding your diet, any restrictions on your activity, and care of your skin and any scars or wounds.

4. Get copies of your hospital records to include in your own medical record and to take with you to each of your physicians' offices. This should include a summary of any injury, illness, disease, or condition diagnosed during the stay; your blood tests, X-rays, and pathology reports; doctors' notes and consultation reports; and your admission history and discharge summary.

5. If you need rehabilitation or other supportive therapy, write down the appointment schedule and where to go.

6. Review your hospital bill carefully to make sure you know what you have been charged for and to identify any charges for services you may not have received. If you need to negotiate a special price for your hospital bill, you should discuss this with the billing department supervisor early in your stay and confirm it again at discharge.

I've just discussed many different pieces of information, any of which could save your life in a hospital, one of the most frightening places in the world. Whenever you are going to enter the hospital, be certain to reread this chapter so these safeguards are fresh in your mind.

## Tips

- Know your nurses, aides, nursing supervisor, pharmacist, and therapists.
- Bring a copy of your medical records and a list of all your medications to the hospital.
- Check your medications each time you receive them.
- Check that your name is on the label of any intravenous fluid or blood transfusion bags.
- Prior to surgery, label the side of your body to be operated on.
- Be certain everyone who touches you washes his or her hands first.
- Know how to call your nurse.
- If you are weak or in pain, use the side rails on your bed and have someone help you when you get up.
- If there are problems, complain immediately.
- When visiting the emergency room, use paramedics for faster care and tell the hospital about any chest pain, arm pain, palpitations, bleeding, fainting, paralysis, or seizure. *Do not minimize any of your symptoms.*
- When you are discharged from the hospital, follow the checklist provided above.

## Today's Medicine and Hospital Care

As health care changes with new reforms, the relationship between hospitals and patients will likely change too. Reduced spending by insurers and the government will reduce staffing at hospitals, so you'll have to be more insistent in getting answers to your questions and attention to your problems. In an effort to reduce costs, many hospitals may merge or join large national networks or chains, resulting in a change in the hospitals' atmospheres, policies, and procedures. Become aware of these changes by reading the newspaper and asking your doctor about them, and think about what impact these cost-saving measures may have on you. Sometimes these mergers or networks can actually enhance the quality of your care, so check on the ratings and evaluations of the new network.

Because some hospitals partner with physicians in health-care delivery systems like accountable-care organizations (ACOs) or medical homes, and other hospitals purchase medical practices, your care coordination may change from the doctor's office to a member of the hospital staff (a nurse practitioner or a disease coordinator such as a diabetes or cardiac care nurse). This individual may help you get more efficient care and avoid hospitalization, but he or she may also try to reduce how much is spent on your care. So be sensitive to whether you are getting the attention or testing you think you need. If you believe you need more care, or if you are not getting better, get a second opinion.

With the increased emphasis on electronic medical records, it is more likely that your hospital has some you will want to read and keep in your own personal health record. Ask the hospital for copies of the doctors' reports (history and physical examinations, consultations, operative notes, pathology reports, radiology reports), lab results, and reports from nutritionists, physical therapists, social services, and respiratory therapists.

Many health-care reforms are focusing on value-based purchasing of hospital and other medical services. This principle applies to paying more for services that provide better value: better outcomes at lower costs. In fact, a requirement for hospitals in the Patient Protection and Affordable Care Act calls for the government to use value-based purchasing when it provides hospital care through Medicare or Medicaid. Under this provision, the government would collect data on health outcomes from hospitals (for example, outcomes after heart attacks or frequency of infections in hospitalized patients), and it would pay more for better outcomes, and less for deficient outcomes. In several years this information would be available to the public, who could use it to choose the right hospital with the best outcomes. This data is not yet available, however, so watch the media to find out when this type of data can be accessed. Even if the legislation is amended, repealed, or annulled, private insurers are focusing reforms on using value-based purchasing.

In order to save money, insurance companies are gradually reducing their payments to hospitals; as a result, many hospitals are dropping contracts with some insurance companies. So regularly check to make sure that the hospitals you have been using are still covered by your insurance. Your insurance plan can provide you with a current list of participating hospitals and physicians, and that type of list changes frequently. Before you register for admission at a hospital, it always pays to double-check to make sure it is still on your insurance plan. If you are too sick to remember, use your family or your advocate to check for you.

Remember, the more changes we see in health-care delivery, the more responsibility you have to make certain you get quality care that is covered by your insurance. Always remain a good "educated consumer" of health care.

# Chapter 19

# Choosing Your Hospital

Some people will tell you that the most important part of your health care is choosing the right hospital. I disagree. A hospital doesn't make your diagnosis or order your tests and treatments—a doctor does. When you need surgery, a hospital doesn't do it—your surgeon does. It is your doctor, not an institution, who cares about you most. But after you have chosen your health plan and then your doctor, you need to decide where you will go if you need an emergency room, surgery, or hospitalization for illness or injury. You must make this choice carefully, and with good recommendations.

Your first and most important source of advice is your primary-care doctor or specialist, who may admit patients to more than one hospital. Ask which hospital the doctor would personally use as a patient, and why. You may choose more than one hospital. The doctor may advise you if there is a hospital that has a particularly good (or bad) track record treating certain conditions. And you may choose a tertiary-care hospital for second opinions (a university hospital, for example). Case in point: one hospital to which I admit patients has excellent cardiac surgery results, and I advise all my cardiology patients to use that hospital. But I send my oncology patients to a different hospital, where the nurses are more attentive and pain is much better controlled. For fast emergency-room care I recommend a third hospital, and for second opinions in medical care, I refer to a university hospital across town.

After seeking your doctor's advice, ask family, friends, other patients, and patient support groups about their experiences. Ask the nurses in your doctor's office which hospital they prefer, or ask other nurses you or your family know—they can be a reliable source of information about the quality of local hospitals. If you have a condition or illness, be sure to ask which hospital is best for that condition, and which hospital is best for emergency care or diagnostic tests.

Once you have narrowed your choice to one or two hospitals, make absolutely sure they are on the list of hospitals covered by your insurance. A call to the insurance company information line (usually listed on the back of your insurance card) will confirm if they are currently contracted. If you have Medicare or Medicaid, call the hospitals to be sure they participate in those programs.

Now you are ready to visit the hospitals to evaluate the patient areas (such as the nursing unit, X-ray department, emergency room, surgical area, and obstetrical and delivery wing), and to assess the general areas, like the waiting rooms and halls, for cleanliness, crowding, and the staff's professional appearance. Inquire at the information desk about hospital tours, which typically are given through the patient-relations office. (Access to many areas of the hospital are usually restricted for patient safety and privacy, so an official tour of those areas is usually required.) Speak to the administrator in charge of patient care to ask about complication and infection rates. Also ask how long patients have to wait in the emergency room before being evaluated.

As you take your tour, what are some of the things you should be looking for? What should you ask nurses, doctors, and patients about? You will be most satisfied if the hospital you choose has courtesy and respect for the patient, offers thorough explanations to patients about their illnesses, and responds rapidly to patients' calls so that pain control is prompt and bedpans are available. The nursing areas should be clean and quiet. Nurses should explain the medicines they give out and provide clear, written instructions upon discharge. If you need an operation or have a serious condition, your hospital should reassure you by providing information about its experience and good outcomes. Do not be turned off if the hospital has a long list of forms you must sign before you are admitted, since that is universal practice.

Tours are useful not only because of what you can see, but also because of what you can ask. So come prepared with your list of concerns—write them down so you do not forget any. Expect direct answers to your questions, or the name of someone who can give you those answers. Write down the name of the person giving the tour, since it's helpful for breaking the ice with others you talk to ("Betty told me I could call you to get an answer to this question…").

You can obtain objective outside evaluations of hospitals from many sources. The most frequently used is undoubtedly the *US News & World Report* annual ranking of American hospitals, which is available online at USNews.com/usnews/health/best-hospitals/tophosp.htm. Only the largest hospitals are ranked, based on evaluations by 180 board-certified physicians, each of whom lists the five hospitals he or she considers best. Factored into this ranking are each hospital's ratio of actual to expected death rates; patient volume; emergency-room capacity; new technology indices; ratio of nurses to beds; and designation (or lack thereof) as a National Cancer Institute cancer center. Because only 180 doctors are polled, it's very possible that this list will miss hospitals in your community, which may also be very good.

There are other rankings as well, which sometimes disagree with *US News & World Report*. These are available through HealthGrades.com, which bases its rankings on national Medicare data and frequency of surgery complications and infections. Your state government may be able to provide additional ratings, which can include risk-adjusted mortality, nursing hours per patient, physician discipline rates, hospital inspection reports, medical malpractice wrongful deaths, and Joint Commission on Accreditation of Healthcare Organizations (JCAHO) hospital accreditation score.

Much of this information can be hard to find and difficult to interpret without the help of a physician or nurse. After reviewing it, ask your doctor about any information that worries you. Only 1 percent of patients who see this type of information change their primary hospital as a result, so if you are having a hard time getting the information, don't worry. But it's good to try so you're more confident about your choice. It's a bit like using a buyer's guide when purchasing a car or appliance—it gives you a good description but no hard-and-fast rules.

Teaching hospitals and university hospitals are often recommended to patients. The advantage of these tertiary-care centers is that they usually have high ratings and provide the most expert care for many serious conditions. The disadvantage involves their size, which can be overwhelming to many patients and families, and which can give an impersonal feel to patient care. "They care about their statistics and their research, but not about me" is a phrase one of my patients used. And emergency services can be surprisingly absent at tertiary facilities, so when considering one, be sure to ask how to get emergency care there.

When using a tertiary-care hospital, you may be assigned a doctor who lacks expertise in your condition unless you have been referred to a specific expert at a university hospital. Very often, most of your immediate care in a tertiary-care or university hospital will be given by an intern, resident, fellow-in-training, or assistant, rather than the expert in charge of your case. More worrisome, if you need an operation, it may be performed by a trainee rather than the board-certified doctor to whom you have been referred.

Therefore, if you are going to receive care at a tertiary teaching hospital, always ask your doctor who will do the surgery, who will give you the anesthesia, and who will make the important day-to-day decisions in your treatment, and ask which consultant or specialist will handle your case. It is always best to be referred to and accepted by a particular physician whom you have selected based on your doctor's advice (or that of others—see chapter 1), rather than just getting the specialist on call for new patients that month. You can and should have a choice in this matter. If you are not given the choice, beware of using that university hospital.

Unless you have a serious condition or illness requiring you to seek out an expert specialist, it's good policy to choose a primary doctor and primary hospital located in your own community for your important day-to-day health care. If you do develop a need for a super-specialist or second opinion, a referral to a good specialist at a highly ranked hospital can be lifesaving. (For more information on choosing a doctor and getting second opinions, see chapters 1 and 15.)

## Tips

- Choose your hospital carefully with the help of doctors, family, friends, and health-care support groups.
- Use the Internet to get patient comments, hospital rankings, and quality reports.
- You should have one or more hospitals on your list for each of these situations: emergency, cardiac, trauma, orthopedic, pediatric, mental health, surgery, general illness, rehabilitation, and second opinions. Review these choices with your doctor.
- Share your choices with your family, who may be the ones bringing you to the hospital when you are sick.

### Contemporary Medicine and Hospital Choices

The times, they are a-changing—and changing fast. A hospital that is good one year may develop problems the next. The reasons vary: a hospital administrator leaves and her replacement has different ideas; a hospital makes new contracts with insurers or physician groups, or hires new doctors; a hospital is plagued by outbreaks of infection; a hospital must reduce staff as a result of declining income; a new hospital wing is built; a nearby hospital closes or another opens, changing the mix of patients. One of my hospitals, listed among the top one hundred during one year, was at risk of closing several years later.

So stay on top of how the hospitals on your list are doing. It's not so hard: your doctor or someone on the hospital staff can give you the inside scoop, you can check the Internet for annual quality checks and report cards, and you can search for patient comments online too. But gone are the old days when your doctor told you to go to the one and only hospital in your area. Now it's up to you to be on top of changes that affect your health care.

# Chapter 20

# "They've Given Up on Me!" Dealing with Chronic Illness in Advanced Stages

Having been trained to care for illness and reverse or halt the progression of disease, doctors generally tend to be most committed to their patients when the patients are responding to treatment. However, sometimes when he can no longer help a patient with chronic, debilitating disease, the doctor becomes frustrated, the patient and the family lose hope and become angry, and the health-care system can seem to "give up" on the patient. The doctor is doing the best he can, but the patient just isn't responding because of the advanced nature of the disease. Although the patient wants to get better, she gets no further advice or encouragement from the physician, who may feel there are no more options. Whether you are a patient or a caregiver, it is important to know that you do have options in this situation.

The first step is to recognize this situation for what it is. Physicians, consultants, or nurses often approach a patient in an advanced stage of chronic disease with certain phrases:

- "There's nothing more I can do."
- "It's just a matter of time."
- "It's time to put your affairs in order."

- "It's time to concentrate on controlling your symptoms and keeping you comfortable."
- "You should consider hospice."
- "Now all we have is palliative-care."

In many of these cases, the physician is correct; there is nothing else that can be done. Often, however, a frustrated physician has failed to consider treatments using newer medications, investigational therapy, more comprehensive symptom control and supportive care, or other modalities that have not been appropriate before. That's the time to get a second opinion to explore all possibilities.

As a patient referred to me from England said, "They've given up on me—and I'm not ready to die." Her widespread breast cancer had failed to respond to two types of chemotherapy, and her English oncologist had no other ideas for treatment that would be paid for by their national health-care system. She came to me for a second opinion. I suggested that the English physicians institute a different program with hormones, new chemotherapy, and a monoclonal antibody. During her excellent two-year remission, the patient was able to go on with her professional singing career throughout the world. So when a fatal prognosis is given, always get another opinion about what can be done.

What results can be obtained from a second opinion given at an advanced stage of chronic illness? You might respond to newer or experimental methods of treatment, combinations of standard treatments plus other modalities, special rehabilitation programs, and/or special supportive-care interventions. In my practice, the results have sometimes been so successful that patients have been able to return to their active lives, working, traveling, or simply enjoying their families. Above all, hope is usually restored, at least for a time.

It is important to be realistic: new therapies at advanced stages of illness are often unsuccessful. However, modern American medicine offers many new treatments that can offer you hope and the possibility of improved function. Find a doctor willing to suggest a new treatment plan if at all possible.

## Palliative-Care Medical Consultations

Palliative-care is a relatively new medical specialty, so many people don't even know what it is. Essentially, palliative specialists help patients control symptoms and adjust to illness. Although most physicians and patients think that palliative-care is appropriate only for patients with a serious chronic illness that is not being treated for cure, this is not the case. Palliative-care can be used across the entire continuum of illness, because severe symptoms and problems adjusting to the stress of illness and therapy can occur anytime, from the initial diagnosis of a disease to its most advanced stages. Palliative-care is typically considered for any patient with symptoms of pain, depression, shortness of breath, or distress that need to be controlled to achieve a better quality of life. Palliative-care physicians frequently provide advice on the effective use of visiting nurses, home-care agencies, in-home help, and hospice, when appropriate. Sometimes palliative-care is considered pre-hospice, or the bridge to hospice care.

For patients facing health care decisions as they approach the end of life, palliative-care specialists can provide valuable guidance and comfort. So if your doctor seems overwhelmed by your illness, consider asking for a palliative-care specialist. And if you're suffering from major stress or depression, think about requesting a psychiatry consultant as well. If pain has become a serious symptom, as often happens in these cases, ask for a pain management specialist to help you improve your quality of life.

You should always expect your doctor to treat your specific symptoms at all times, during any disease. If the doctor is not treating your symptoms (pain, depression, anxiety, fatigue, weight loss, or any problem causing you distress), ask for a second opinion or a palliative-care consultation. If your community hospital does not have a palliative-care specialist or palliative-care center, ask for a referral to a larger tertiary-care center or university where such resources are available.

## Hospice: When Further Therapy Won't Work or Isn't Wanted

When all your doctors and second opinions agree that there is no further active therapy that would reverse or control your disease, or when you simply do not want any more treatments, hospice can improve your symptoms and relieve your suffering. Either in the home or in an inpatient setting (nursing homes, hospitals, or free-standing hospice centers), hospice nurses and volunteers can deliver great benefits to patients and their families, relieving much of the stress of end-of-life care and decision making.

## Choosing a Hospice

In the past, patients in a hospice program could receive no further active anticancer therapy (no chemotherapy or radiation treatments). Now, however, many hospice programs allow patients to get some treatments, such as short-course radiation therapy or low-cost chemotherapy, to relieve symptoms. Since this policy varies according to the program, you need to ask your hospice provider if treatments to control the underlying illness can be continued if needed.

The number of hospices in the United States has increased because health-care programs have increased funding for hospice care. The majority of the forty-eight thousand American hospices are now for-profit programs, and their quality varies. Many hospices are not certified by Medicare, so be certain to ask if the program you're considering is certified. (If it is, it's probably among the higher-quality programs.) Ask your physicians too, about the quality of the hospice program you are considering.

Usually, insurance will pay for hospice only if the patient's life expectancy is less than six months. However, doctors are not perfect at estimating length of life, so in most cases a patient with advanced disease of any kind can be eligible for hospice if any doctor says it is likely that the patient will survive less than six months. In many hospices, at least a few patients with slowly progressing illnesses have stayed there a year or two, or even longer. So be sure to ask if your insurance will cover extended hospice care if your disease advances more slowly than predicted.

For help evaluating hospice programs and learning about them in more detail, visit the website of the National Hospice and Palliative-Care Organization, NHPCO.org, and check the section called "Caring Connections." The site is very user-friendly and offers plenty of good information to familiarize you with hospice programs.

Medicare-insured patients who have elected to receive hospice care should be aware of the fact that they can go off hospice care up to three times to receive standard care, including hospitalization, antibiotics, chemotherapy, surgery, or radiation therapy. Once a Medicare patient enters hospice for the fourth time, however, he or she cannot discontinue it again without losing the hospice benefit. Of course, most patients who enter hospice never leave the program.

Ask your doctor if you are nearing this point in your illness, and ask which hospices are available in your area. To determine which program would be best for you, ask all your doctors, talk to the hospice nurses, and visit the hospice inpatient areas. Talk to families of other patients who have been recently cared for by the hospice staff (the program can provide you with names and contact information). The sincerity and experience of most hospice staff and physician hospice directors facilitate the process of making all the important choices and arrangements regarding end-of-life issues.

At the end stages of illness, hospice can make uncomfortable and frightening life transitions more comfortable and dignified. So let your physician know when you're ready to discuss hospice services. Be aware that for patients with diseases like cancer, the typical length of life on a hospice program is usually brief. A longer life on hospice is more typical in patients with slower-progressing diseases, such as Alzheimer's, AIDS, stroke, cardiac failure, and emphysema. Shop carefully to be certain you choose a hospice that is comfortable for you.

## Euthanasia

The trail-blazing experience with euthanasia in Oregon has taught physicians about symptoms at the end of life. Since pain is patients' most feared symptom, one would expect that pain would be the most frequent reason to request euthanasia. But surprisingly, very few of the patients wanting euthanasia in Oregon had uncontrolled pain; most were suffering from severe depression. Many also were experiencing unstable support at home, especially caregiver problems. Sometimes the patient was simply afraid of being a burden for the caregiver (typically a family or friend). But more often, the severity of the patient's distress and symptoms and the amount of work required to care for him or her had produced caregiver "burnout"—soon followed by patients giving up and wanting euthanasia.

So as your disease progresses or the end of life approaches, talk to your physician about how to recognize depression-related symptoms and whether you need antidepression medicines. Pain control should always be a high priority, both to avoid discomfort and to prevent depression. This can allow better quality of life, more satisfactory interactions with family and friends, and less stress on your caregiver.

Look for and address symptoms of caregiver fatigue or burnout. Many medical centers have caregiver respite programs through which patients can be admitted to a hospital or hospice, allowing caregivers to readjust (commonly referred to as a time to "recharge the batteries").

## Tips

- Recognize the signs that your doctor has run out of treatments. (Often the physician will just tell you directly.)
- If you feel your physicians have given up on you, and you still want to fight the illness, consider a second opinion.
- Look into other important sources of suggestions for new treatments: patient groups; nurses; the National Institutes of Health; physician associations such as the American Society of Clinical Oncology for cancer and the American Society of Hematology for blood diseases; or disease-oriented organizations such as the American Cancer Society, the American Heart Association, and the American Diabetes Association.
- Consider asking for a referral to a specialist at a university hospital.
- When there is nothing else that can be done, request a palliative-care specialist and consider whether hospice is appropriate for you.
- Recognize any uncontrolled symptoms, request treatment for them, and be aware of caregiver burnout.

## Today's Medicine and Care Approaching End of Life

Health-care reform is most concerned about controlling the escalating costs of health care—and those costs are significant for patients in advanced stages of illness, especially in the six months preceding death. This fact has led health-care economists and governmental advisers to recommend the earlier use of hospice and more limited use of treatments near the end of life.

Influenced by these opinions, your physician may suggest that you abandon further care efforts. He may be reluctant to order tests, procedures, surgery, or expensive treatments because you have not responded to prior treatment or you have relapsed (which is common in cancer therapy).

More worrisome, your health plan may have restrictive guidelines about how much therapy should be approved. For example, some insurance plans suggest no more than two types of chemotherapy for lung cancer should be approved, even if the patient is feeling well and wants additional treatment. In those situations, you have to be proactive, insisting on a second opinion about further care. Referrals to hospice without consideration of additional treatments is not uncommon in managed-care situations, such as HMOs or ACOs, where the health plan or physicians may be at risk for paying for additional expensive therapy. Be cautious in such situations.

The 2010 Patient Protection and Affordable Care Act has an interesting provision. Although traditional hospice programs will not pay for chemotherapy even if it is designed to relieve symptoms, under the Affordable Care Act, children with cancer can receive chemotherapy treatments paid for by Medicaid, even if they are enrolled in hospice. This provision should help these young patients get relief for their symptoms, as well as life-prolonging therapy. I hope other insurers will follow this policy in the future.

If your chronic illness is progressing, talk to your doctor about your prognosis, realistic expectations for your longevity and quality of life, and all the health-care options available to you.

# Chapter 21

# "I'm Overwhelmed!"
# Coping with Prolonged Treatments

So many tests, so many treatments, so many medicines—chronic illness is overwhelming to many patients. With medical and scientific progress resulting in a longer average life expectancy, treatment programs have become longer-lasting, harder to endure, more expensive, and accompanied by more side effects. Treatments often require much more of your time and effort to get through compared to previous eras, when medicine had so little to offer that therapies were simpler.

My patients often say, "How am I ever going to get through this?" Indeed, you may have asked that same question yourself.

The most important step you can take is to decide that, starting now, you will have a positive attitude toward your life, and you will do whatever's necessary to preserve and enjoy it. Making this commitment means telling yourself that you are now going to change: you will now see every glass as half-full, not half-empty.

Write down this promise as a reminder to focus on the bright side of your life. Then write your personal goals and the activities that are most important to you (your "bucket list"). When you stay focused on those objectives, you will consider any medical treatments, tests, or appointments not as barriers or burdens, but as necessary vehicles to get you where you want to go.

I once asked a friend who had survived muscle cancer surgery and chemotherapy what kept him going, what enabled him to accept all his months of treatments. "Doc, I just made a new life plan," he said. "I told myself that from now on, my plan was to wake up tomorrow healthy, happy, and smiling. And I have, ever since, even when I had tough things to do." And every time I see him, he's happy, smiling, and working to enjoy every minute of every day.

But if you're struggling to try to cope with a serious illness and the constant pressure of treatment after treatment, you might find that a project—whether it's a trip, family event, reunion, or diary—will help redirect your focus from your medical care to a world of personal goals. One of my patients decided to make a film about his treatment, and the project helped relieve his anxiety and improve his depression.

Another patient developed a unique project to reduce her depression. She went to her business, a little bookstore, and set out two chairs. She called them the "laughing chairs" and invited her customers to sit down and chat—but they had to be smiling and upbeat and tell jokes or funny stories. Well, her attitude improved, her depression disappeared, and both she and her customers felt better as a result. You may not have a bookstore, but you can try the laughing-chair technique to improve your conversations with your family and friends. Since so many patients with chronic debilitating illness face progressive isolation from friends and then family, any activity that increases visits and facilitates conversation about nonmedical topics is most useful.

One of my patients decided to develop a more positive attitude by reading only humorous books, watching comedies, and listening to jokes. You might want to give that a try, focusing on upbeat, empowering books and movies.

Another of my patients decided he wanted to make a movie about his personal struggle to overcome lung cancer. As a psychologist who had made many educational films in his field, he felt that a film about his treatments would help others. He received all his standard treatments, radiation, clinical trial therapy, and supportive medicines as a film crew followed him around at home and in our center. This project helped him and his family keep a positive attitude and bear up under the symptoms and pressures of his advanced cancer care. After many months, he passed away. At the premier of his movie—which became the film *One Man's Fight for Life*, still shown periodically on HBO—his family told me how helpful the project had been to him, and how they felt it would help others as well. In a medical crisis, documenting your journey on paper, in photos, or on film can help your family and others, and it may just give you the spirit to carry on.

## What Helps Patients Get Through Their Illness

Because I wanted to understand what had helped my patients get through their cancer chemotherapy, I asked them to complete a survey to identify and rate those resources. Their answers surprised me.

Only a few patients gave a very high rating to patient support groups (generally organized by hospitals or health-care organizations like the American Cancer Society, with information at Cancer.org, and the Cancer Support Community, with online support and referrals to local groups at CancerSupportCommunity.org). On an individual basis, and especially with younger patients and patients who communicate well with others in a group setting, these support groups do help by providing a social environment where they can solve problems and get suggestions regarding their care. Some patients reported that when another patient took a turn for the worse, it was depressing and stressful.

The highest-rated sources of support were religion and family and friends. Faith and talking to religious leaders helped keep many patients from giving up. Others were empowered by the support of family or friends who kept up their spirits, provided motivation, and refused to be discouraged by the illness.

You should learn from these patients. Their struggles may be the same as yours. And their methods for getting through the needed tests and treatments can be resources you can use too, to help you survive.

## Resources for Chronic Care

The number of Internet resources for the chronically ill has grown exponentially. Both government websites (CDC.gov and HHS. gov) and private free sites (WebMD.com, MayoClinic.com, CancerSupportCommunity.org, CancerCare.org, or HealthLine.com) can suggest ways to focus your inner strengths toward healing rather than suffering. You or a family member or friend should use this online information to help make positive decisions in your chronic care.

## Tips

- Choose a treatment in which you have high confidence, and a physician whom you trust.
- Use patient support groups for encouragement.
- Get the positive support of your family or friends. Avoid family and friends who give you only negative feedback.
- Set goals (like a celebration or a trip) as a key to getting through a tough program of treatment.
- Use your religion and religious leaders to give you support.
- Consider setting a mission for yourself; find meaning in your struggle.

## Contemporary Medicine and Fighting Illness

One of the changes brought by health-care reform is increased use of care coordinators. Usually nurse practitioners, these individuals can suggest support mechanisms that can help sustain you through difficult times. But be aware that due to cost concerns, there is also pressure to give less treatment to chronically ill patients and push them instead into palliative and hospice care. By working with your physician, you can make realistic plans for your care, with realistic expectations about the outcome.

# Section 3:
# Caring and Advocating for Others

# Chapter 22

## Caring for Children

When you plan to become a parent, your commitment to health and wellness takes on added significance. The realization that health is necessary for the entire family, from conception to old age, and that it is your responsibility to begin that process yourself, should lead you to become more serious about your health care and your doctor's advice.

Of course, children need to be healthy too. But they cannot commit to healthy practices for themselves, as you, an adult, can do. Quite to the contrary, they depend totally on you, the parent, to be their designated health advocate and to make all the correct decisions for them. You have the obligation to dedicate yourself to healthy practices, both for them and for you.

The principles of health care for your children are similar to those I've already outlined for your own health, but with slight changes in focus and sources of information. In general, you must seek out the highest-quality health care available to you, get insurance that enables your child to have excellent pediatric services, and find the right doctor for both you and your children. And you should start as soon as you decide to get pregnant.

## A Parenting Plan

When considering getting pregnant, talk to your primary-care physician about healthy practices that promote pregnancy. Be sure that your lifestyle includes a good diet, exercise, and vitamins. Avoiding unhealthy behaviors like smoking and drinking can reduce the risk of fetal loss (spontaneous abortion) and fetal abnormalities (malformations and poor fetal growth). As soon as a pregnancy is discovered, commit yourself totally to quality health care for your new baby. Following the tips in chapter 25 on health insurance, find the best health plan you can afford to cover your child's health.

Once you or your partner is pregnant, choose an obstetrician and begin prenatal care. Refer to the advice in chapter 1 on how to choose a doctor, and remember the most important advice: ask your primary doctor for a referral to an obstetrician whom he would personally use to deliver his own child. At your first visit with the obstetrician, obtain all the information the office has available about caring for your pregnancy, and ask the doctor to recommend childbirth and parenting programs.

Begin to evaluate which hospital you will select for delivery. Since this is a very important decision, start by asking the obstetrician for a recommendation. Then, in keeping with the advice in chapter 19 on how to choose a hospital, ask the most important questions, like "Would you use this hospital to have your own baby?" Once you have a good recommendation from the doctor, take a prenatal tour of the chosen hospital. Evaluate the delivery area to be sure you are comfortable with the level of care, attentiveness of the staff, and cleanliness of the environment. Review with your doctor the quality of the neonatal ICU, where the health-care team would take care of any severe complications in your baby. Ask the hospital or your physician about classes in labor, delivery, and parenting for you and your partner.

Decide in consultation with your obstetrician whether an anesthesiologist will be used in your delivery, and check the quality of that physician with your doctor and others. Again, the chapter on choosing a doctor will help you.

Select a pediatrician before your baby is born. Your first source of information should be your own family. Ask them about their experiences, and then discuss those experiences with your obstetrician and primary physician.

Review chapter 1 on choosing a doctor, and ask your obstetrician the important questions about whom the doctor would personally choose as a pediatrician and why. Then visit the pediatrician's office to look around and evaluate where your child will be getting checkups and care. Since networking is always important, ask others in the waiting room about their experiences with the pediatrician's care and the pediatric nurses.

When you have a newborn, will you and your partner both be confident in your parenting skills? So that you are prepared even before delivery, ask your pediatrician about parenting resources, including parenting classes. Learn about emergency procedures for your baby, like infant Heimlich maneuver and infant CPR.

Once you have delivered, check with your pediatrician about keeping on schedule for "well-baby visits" and vaccinations. Ask the doctor's office to recommend websites and books for learning the additional skills you will need as your baby matures.

Start a medical health record for your newborn. This is important for tracking healthy growth and recognizing and solving problems as they arise. See appendix 1 for an outline of a personal medical record you can use as a template.

As your children grow, evaluate them for unhealthy habits. With your pediatrician, develop a plan to correct any problems and prevent later illness—and then implement the plan. If your child is not improving, discuss the problem with the doctor and get a second opinion if necessary. Remember to take a list of questions with you!

Mentor your children: you should always set good examples in lifestyle and habits such as diet, exercise, medical checkups, prompt attention to problems or symptoms, and preventing illness. Ask and receive the advice of your primary-care physician whenever you are uncertain about an aspect of your child's health. Create a safe home environment, and develop an emergency plan for the family. Make sure your child always feels loved, and always plan your day so you can spend unrushed and uninterrupted time with your child.

## Sources of Detailed Information

Most obstetricians' and pediatricians' offices can provide you with a set of parenting guides. But sometimes these offices are more focused on checkups and vaccinations than on giving you the resources you need to have day-to-day confidence as a parent. Fortunately, there are plenty of good parenting resources online to start you out on improving your well-baby plan. Here are my recommendations for getting the latest information from the Internet. Always check what you've learned with your pediatrician.

The very best of the best for general parenting advice is the website of the American Academy of Pediatrics. It is comprehensive, supplementing what your own doctor has said and providing ideas to discuss with her at your child's next office visit. Go to AAP.org/parents and then click on the link for your child's age. Particularly useful is the "family readiness list" to provide a safe home environment.

Other valuable websites for parents:

- CDC.gov/women/owh/kids/abc.htm (a government website)
- FamilyDoctor.org/children.html (informative articles)
- KidsHealth.org (physician-approved information)
- ChildParenting.about.com (parenting guide and newsletter)
- AllThatWomenWant.com/parentingwebguide.htm (guide to help both baby and mother)
- GuideOurChildren.com (useful online book)
- TheNewParentsGuide.com (product and shopping information)

Wanting to be well prepared to care for their children from prenatal times on, most parents have medical guidebooks at home. These two are particularly useful:

- *Caring for your Baby and Young Child, Revised Edition, Birth to Age 5*, edited by Stephen P. Shelov, MD, FAAP, and Robert E Hammermann, MD, FAAP (Bantam Books, 1998)
- *The American Academy of Pediatrics Guide to Your Child's Symptoms: The Official, Complete Home Reference, Birth*

*Through Adolescence*, edited by Donald Schiff, MD, FAAP, and Stephen P. Shelov, MD, FAAP (Villard Books, 1997)

As advocates of more unusual ideas about parenting, William and Martha Sears introduced concepts helpful to many parents with *The Baby Book: Everything You Need to Know about Your Baby from Birth to Age 2*. Review their recommendations with your own doctor before trying them.

## Tips

- Prepare for pregnancy before getting pregnant. In consultation with your primary physician, choose an obstetrician and maintain the best health habits.
- As soon as you or your partner becomes pregnant, visit an obstetrician and begin prenatal care. Choose the best hospital for delivery, and follow the best prenatal health plan to minimize fetal problems. Get more prenatal information from the Internet and published sources.
- Select a pediatrician with the help of your primary physician and obstetrician.
- Consider attending parenting classes and parent support groups.
- Start a medical health record for your newborn.
- Mentor your children, give them love and attention, and share healthy lifestyle habits to set them on a course for success.

## Today's Medicine and Baby and Child Care

Universal commitment to the health and welfare of babies and children underlies many of the health-care changes that are occurring each year. Federally legislated changes have increased the availability of Medicaid resources for children in indigent or low-income families. With increased numbers of HMOs and new funding of pediatric patient ACOs, more programs are available for prenatal care and for infants and children. These include "well-baby" programs, preventive health services, and improved access for symptom care. Although we will continue to see increased use of managed-care systems, all health-care organizations will be required to report outcomes and comply with recommended preventive care services. That mandate will help ensure that managed care systems give increasingly high-quality health care for children.

# Chapter 23

## Caring for the Elderly

Elderly people face different challenges than other adults—challenges that must be addressed or their quality and length of life deteriorate. Of course, that is the reason geriatric medicine was developed as a medical specialty: to improve the care of aging individuals. If you care for an elderly family member, what can you do to maintain and improve his or her health?

Perhaps the first question we should ask is, when does a person who is just older become "elderly," requiring special care? Geriatric care should be considered as soon as any symptoms of aging become apparent. These include memory loss, unsteadiness of gait, difficulty with self-care, eating disorders, sleep disturbances, reduced vision and hearing, and mental-psychological challenges. When any of these symptoms occurs, you should visit a primary-care physician with the older person and ask the physician to develop a plan addressing them. (Once these problems develop, they can worsen rapidly.) Ask whether a geriatric medicine specialist might be appropriate.

A geriatric specialist often conducts special tests to detect symptoms and assess function. These tests can include ADL (Activities of Daily Living), IADL (Instrumental Activities of Daily Living), sleep studies, cognitive and memory testing, tests for depression and distress, and gait evaluation. Other specialists may also be needed, such as pulmonologists for sleep disorders; neurologists for loss of motor skills, movement disorder (tremor), cognitive impairment, or memory loss; orthopedists for gait disorders; and cardiologists for heart failure.

A patient's health-care plan and medical team change when he or she enters geriatric care. The patient's family can help with this transition by asking questions of the primary doctor and facilitating the testing and specialist consultations so important in developing the proper treatment plan.

The website RealAge.com is helpful for evaluating a geriatric patient's "biological age." By asking detailed questions about an individual, the website can determine if the person is biologically older than his chronological age (and therefore likely to have a more limited life expectancy and require immediate medical attention), or biologically younger and likely to have a longer-than-average life.

## A New Look at Resources

Those who care for the elderly must have resources that are different from those of other caregivers. Their experts should be skilled in improving or maintaining the health, function, and quality of life of both the patient and his or her caregivers (family and friends). Being a caregiver for an elderly patient is a tough job, and finding the best resources and support makes the outcome better and happier. Challenges can become accomplishments, work can become team goals and activities, and frustration can become satisfaction.

The best resource for the caregiver is the primary-care physician, internist, or geriatrician who leads the team, creates and evaluates the plan, and orders the support testing and treatments. Information is also available online from the American Association of Family Physicians at AAFP.org and from the American Geriatric Society at its website, AmericanGeriatrics. org (see the section on education for caregivers) and in its publication, *Eldercare at Home.*

Keeping an elderly patient fit and at home, and therefore decreasing the need for emergency-room visits and hospitalization, is an important challenge. The longer a patient is in the hospital, the higher the likelihood of needing nursing-home care and the greater the risk of chronic infection with antibiotic-resistant bacteria. The best solution is having an outpatient case manager (or "care coordinator"), who can keep closer tabs on all the problems challenging the elderly patient and coordinate all specialist and home-nursing care. This can minimize the need for hospitalization. Information about finding and using this type of support can be found through the National Association of Professional Geriatric Case Managers at CaseManager.com. Home-nursing care is also important as a support to minimize physician, laboratory, and emergency-room visits. Learn more about this category of service through the website of the Visiting Angels, a home-based care network, at VisitingAngels.com.

Rehabilitation services can be necessary to help the elderly maintain their function at home. Physical therapy helps with gait and mobility problems, occupational therapy helps with activities of daily living, and speech therapy can help with swallowing disorders and communication difficulties. There are also sleep programs, which can restore adequate sleep patterns. Psychologists can help with common geriatric problems such as cognitive dysfunction and depression.

Social workers at the hospital can help marry the patient's need for resources with his or her insurance plan coverage. You can discuss the benefits of assisted living and the later necessity for skilled nursing-home support not only with the patient's physician, but also with the social worker, who can refer you to assisted-living facilities and nursing homes for your evaluation.

The doctor is key to the patient's health care, setting up a plan for the coordinators and ancillary medical support. Be sure to ask about each of these support systems; the more support the patient and caregiver have, the less likely the need for a transition to out-of-home living.

One of the toughest challenges for the elderly is continuing activities that give them satisfaction and quality of life. Their prior social systems change—or, in the words of my ninety-three-year old patient, "All my friends have just plain died. There's no one left to have any fun with." As a family, create opportunities for "fun" by hosting celebrations involving the elderly in planning and gifting, creating legacies, developing family history projects like photo albums or recorded stories, getting a small dog or cat, and having more outings and vacations together.

## Tips

- Be aware of new challenges for family members older than fifty.
- Discuss any problems with the patient's primary physician. Develop a plan and implement it.
- Consider geriatric consultation.
- Use a case manager or coordinator with the guidance of the patient's physician.
- Develop a comprehensive support system for the patient.
- Diligently read information about geriatric care on the Internet and discuss it with the care team.

## Today's Medicine and Elder Care

Health-care reform recognizes the aging of the American population. Key changes are coming through government regulations and private insurance programs to help the elderly remain functional and healthy and reduce the need for hospitalization, primarily by offering more preventive services and paying physicians more for care coordination. This increases the availability of nurse practitioners, care coordinators, and support systems for geriatric patients.

But these changes also increase your responsibility to ask for these resources during ever-shorter office visits with the physician. If you are attentive to your elderly family member's emerging health care needs, you can take advantage of these newly covered services at the earliest possible time.

# Chapter 24

# Caring for the Infirmed

By age ninety-three, Fay had developed heart failure, Alzheimer's disease, diabetes, and arthritis. Although she lived at home with her daughter and son-in-law, she needed round-the-clock in-home health care and frequent physician visits, and her complex medication schedule required constant attention from her caregivers. "You can't believe how hard it is to keep her at home and out of the nursing home. I'm mentally and physically exhausted, and it's costing me a fortune," said her daughter Linda. With Linda's help, Fay lived another two years, enjoying love and attention at home and celebrating birthdays and anniversaries together with her family, with only two short stays in the hospital for infections. How did Linda do it? Could you do what she did?

When a serious chronic condition afflicts a patient, infirmity can occur—and it can occur at any age, although it often overlaps with being elderly. The characteristics of infirmity are physical or mental ailment, bodily disability with weakness and frailty, and usually an inability to care for oneself; an infirmed person requires the care of a family member or friend in order to live at home and maintain function. Infirmity can happen suddenly and unexpectedly: a formerly active person suffers a stroke or heart attack, or she has an accident that leaves her with a physical disability. Where else besides family can someone like this turn for help? If you're asked to be a caregiver, how can you respond?

## Getting the Right Physicians

Successfully dealing with a disability requires having the right doctors on the patient's health care team. If the patient who has suffered fractures with trauma requires not only orthopedic care, but also good primary care, a physiatrist (rehabilitation specialist), and possibly a pain specialist, together with nutrition support, rehabilitation therapy, home care, appropriate durable medical equipment, and often psychological support. A patient with heart failure needs not only a primary-care doctor, but also a cardiologist and cardiac-rehabilitation services, possibly a dietician, psychologist, and home-care services, and sometimes an endocrinologist (for diabetic care and metabolic syndrome). With lung cancer, patients need not only an oncologist, but also the primary-care physician, a pulmonologist, a lung surgeon, a pain specialist, nutrition support, and respiratory and rehabilitation therapy, and often palliative-care. But disabled patients are incapable of asking for all the support they need or ensuring that they receive it.

This is where you come in. Family members (or friends) are essential for keeping up with the care plan designed by the lead physician and complying with the patient's requirements for medication, treatments, supportive-care visits, rehabilitation, and emotional support. Often, one caregiver is not enough—it may not take a village, but it certainly takes an entire support team, plus family and friends. Making sure all the patient's needs are met is essential to good outcomes, and the disabled patient is often unable to convey those needs to all the doctors on his or her health-care team. Finding the right doctors for that team, as well as requesting consultations and necessary supportive care, are challenges you, the caregiver, can meet.

## How to Get All Needed Care

Begin with some questions for the patient's primary doctor: What other doctors could help the patient get better faster? What supportive care can you order to help recovery and help me deal with the illness? Do we need home care? What support can we get at home to keep the patient outside the hospital? Is a care coordinator available, or can someone in your office take on that role?

Understanding the prognosis is crucial to having realistic expectations about outcomes. Not only must the doctor set appropriate, achievable goals, but you and other family members must fully understand those goals to avoid frustration and conflict. If some caregivers' expectations are too high, tension and anger will arise. To reduce that possibility and get everyone on the same page, organize family conferences. Enlist the help of care coordinators and social workers, who can help identify misunderstandings and reconcile family issues.

The doctor can help too, by identifying specific risks the patient may face. For example, treating trauma patients means keeping them safe from falls and reinjury. Treating cancer patients means avoiding infections, the most frequent cause of hospitalization and death. So you need to ask the doctor, "What are the common risks the patient faces, and how can we prevent them? What is the prognosis for cure, for recovery, for control, for stability, or for deterioration? How long will the patient live? Will hospitalization be needed? If so, how can we be sure any hospital stays are brief?"

## Care for the Caregiver

Caregiving is not easy; it's no coincidence that the incidence of stress, fatigue, and even frank illness in caregivers is high. As a caregiver, you need support too.

That is the reason to put together the best team possible to help the patient. More hands mean less work for the individual caregiver and more shared responsibility.

Sharing these concerns with the doctor, care coordinator, social workers, and home-health nurses is very important. The master plan for patient care should include being aware of your own risks as caregiver and incorporating ways to avoid overwork, stress, and physical illness. Ask the doctor, "Can taking care of the patient make me sick? How can I prevent getting ill? How can I stay healthy enough to continue to help the patient? What do I do if I need more support? If I need some time off, will you help me get it, and how?" Knowing how to take a "time-out" will give you the confidence to be a better caregiver.

## Resources

Advice for caregivers for any infirmed patient can be found through the disease-specific resources listed in chapter 5 on using the Internet. But there is other helpful information online too, including AARP's caregiver suggestions at AARP.org/relationships/caregiving, advice through the Alzheimer's Disease Research link at AHAF.org, information from the Cancer Support Community at CancerSupportCommunity.org, and the website of Caring Connections, CaringInfo.org.

Sometimes caregivers need more support than their existing network provides. There are individuals who sell their services as caregiver coaches; you can usually find them through social workers or home-care coordinators who are sources of information about the resources in your own community. Most physicians are not familiar with these services, however. Once you have found a coach, be sure to get personal references before hiring them. With sick patients, unfortunately, sometimes the only workable solution is a skilled nursing facility, a hospital-centered palliative-care program, or even hospice, if therapy is not working.

## Tips

- An extensive, comprehensive professional team is necessary to care for an infirmed patient. Your doctor can help set this up, but be sure to ask for all possible help.
- Be sure your caregiver team is large and committed.
- Address the challenges that you, as a caregiver, will be facing.

## Today's Health Care and Patient Caregivers

Insurers and government now recognize the need for family caregivers. Reforms and additional programs have been developed to ensure that insurance plans cover more support services; some state programs (like Medicaid) actually pay for family-provided home-care services. Check with your physician and social worker to see what your plan covers.

To replace expensive in-hospital care, HMOs and PPOs (as well as newly formed ACOs) are paying physicians to provide care coordination for many chronic illnesses. Hospital programs have stepped in as well, by adding caseworkers or coordinators to many of their center-based programs (cardiac, lung, diabetes, or orthopedic programs, for example). So be sure to check with your doctor and hospital to see what sort of care coordination they offer, and see if nearby tertiary-care centers offer programs (and care coordination) specific to your family member's disease.

As Americans live longer, the number of chronically ill patients will grow, along with their health care needs. Because reducing health-care costs depends on more effective support programs for the chronically ill, these programs will continue to grow and develop. If a program is not available for you today, don't give up—ask again in two or three months.

Section 4:

# Insuring and Financing Your Health Care

# Chapter 25

# Finding Health Insurance and a Broker

Stop right now and think about your health insurance. This is the freakiest part of being able to survive with American medicine: the decision you make about your health insurance is the most critical decision you will make in getting great health care and living as long as possible. Why? Because which health plan you choose determines which doctors and hospitals you can use, how often you can use them, and whether you stay in charge of your health.

Because of the high cost of medicine, you need some type of health insurance. When you go to a doctor for a routine checkup or a mild complaint like a cold or a bladder infection, the cost is not very high. But if you become seriously sick, your medical costs can quickly rise to tens or even hundreds of thousands of dollars. Therefore, choosing the best insurance you can afford is one of the most important health decisions you can make.

## Why You Absolutely Need Some Type of Health Insurance

There are still some individuals who think that since they are healthy today, they can just wait until they are sick or elderly to get insurance. Unfortunately, there are two problems with this strategy: First, trauma can happen at any time, and whether it's a car accident, a fall at home, or an injury during a vacation, you cannot anticipate it. Second, at least one of every three Americans has one or more chronic conditions—and one of six Americans has two or more. Every chronic condition, even in its earliest stages, can require expensive medicine to control symptoms and prevent progression. This can cost a fortune.

As you try to understand the costs of health care, the first thing you should know is that doctors and hospitals have two prices. The highest price is the usual or customary charge. This is the full retail price, like the sticker price on a new car, and it may be several times higher than the price negotiated by an insurance company. Remember, if you do not have insurance, or if you are receiving care outside your health plan, you will have to pay this high charge, and if you don't, the doctor or hospital may even send a collection agency after you.

The lower price, like the discounted price you bargain for when buying a new car, is the allowable charge (also called the "covered charge") for which your insurance company has contracted on your behalf with the doctor, hospital, or laboratory. It is usually a small fraction of the retail charge. So the important rule to be learned is this: always have insurance to limit how much you will have to pay, and always make sure you are receiving care from a doctor or hospital contracted with (participating in) your health plan. This rule also applies to pharmacies, medical supplies from durable medical equipment stores or agencies, home-nursing agencies, physical therapists, radiology and imaging centers, pathologists who interpret biopsies, hospitals to which you are referred, and specialists for second opinions. If you don't follow this rule, you can quickly go broke.

The only way you can escape paying "retail" for medical care is to have some type of insurance. So the question for you isn't whether to get insurance, but what kind of insurance you want and can afford.

A patient of mine brought her $60,000 hospital visit bill to my office, worried she would have to declare bankruptcy, until I pointed out to her that since she had PPO insurance, she did not owe $60,000. In fact, the allowed charge on her plan was only $15,000, and she was required to pay just 20 percent of the allowed charge, or $3,000. (Although she was relieved, I warned her to object to any bill she received that asked her for more than $3,000. Very often, hospitals, medical offices, labs, and radiology units mistakenly bill more that the allowable co-payment mandated by the insurance contract.) Because my patient had insurance, her bill and out-of-pocket expense were much less than "retail," and through her insurance company's help line she could review her bill for excess charges.

## My Best Advice

Although I will discuss each type of health insurance in great detail, I'm going to start the discussion by giving you my best advice up-front, so you can keep it in mind as you read the rest of this chapter.

If you are over age sixty-five, I strongly recommend enrolling in Medicare and having a secondary insurance (also called a Medicare supplemental or "Medigap" policy). If you do not have many financial assets, consider obtaining Medicare with Medicaid as secondary insurance, but remember that you must qualify for Medicaid financially.

If you are under sixty-five, I strongly urge you to obtain PPO insurance. If you can't afford it, consider establishing a medical savings account or using an HMO with a point-of-service (POS) option.

## How to Find a Health-Insurance Broker

When you are considering life insurance, you can get valuable advice from a life-insurance broker. When you need disability insurance, again you can get help from a broker. In the same way, a health-insurance broker specializes can help you assess all your options for health insurance. He or she can make sure you don't make a mistake in getting the right insurance for your needs and your bank account.

Regardless of your age, a good health-insurance agent is a valuable resource. You may have to use this agent again and again, since sources of your insurance may periodically change. As continuing health-care reforms change the rules, benefits, and costs of insurance, an agent can help you choose the appropriate health plan. I call my health-insurance agent at least once a year to ask new questions and get updated advice.

You can ask your family or friends about the agent they use, but you can also go online to get a list of names in your area. Try visiting the National Association of Health Underwriters at NAHU.org or the Association of Health Insurance Advisors at AHIA.net. To get a general idea of health insurance rates, visit InsuranceTracker.com. Other good resources are the National Association of Insurance Commissioners at NAIC.org (which lists complaints about any insurance company), eHealthInsurance.com, or HealthInsuranceInfo.net.

Is this health insurance stuff expensive? Undoubtedly it is. However, there is nothing worse than the frustration of not being able to obtain therapy that may help you avoid a chronic disability—or that may even save your life—when your health insurance is too restrictive or you don't have any insurance at all. A broker can help you through the daunting task of comparing plans and benefits and costs. Use this wise counsel and consider your options very carefully before you enter into a commitment for insurance! You get only one body—insure it well.

## Where to Start

Since choosing an insurance plan can be the most confusing part of health-care decisions, the following sections are designed to help you with that choice by comparing different types of plans. But the following descriptions are also short. While they'll put the options into some perspective for you, don't make a decision until you study actual plans that are given to you by Medicare, Medicare supplemental insurers, or PPO or HMO plans. Although reviewing an actual policy is quite tedious, some of the principles below can help you focus on the most important points and ask the right questions.

But whom do you ask? Who is there to help you? Many people are paralyzed when facing this decision, even to the point of not choosing any insurance and leaving themselves vulnerable to potentially fatal consequences. But you won't be overwhelmed if you realize how many resources you actually have.

While many people try to hide when they know an insurance agent is nearby, health insurance is one area where some of the best advice is both readily available and free. Because there are so many types of insurance policies, discuss your options with an agent who has experience selling health insurance; many agents have considerable expertise in this area. (To find an agent, see the online resources listed earlier in this chapter.) An experienced insurance agent can advise you about various plans and walk you through comparable coverage at different costs. Frequently the agent can relate others' experiences with a particular plan, describing any problems and frustrations. An agent also can verify that a particular plan is licensed in your state—critical to receiving covered care from local doctors and hospitals.

At work, you can contact the human-resources department for recommendations, but remember that they may have been instructed to push certain plans above others for cost reasons. At the doctor's office, you can get advice from the insurance coordinator or office manager about which plans are accepted and which work well. At the hospital, ask the insurance clerk about the different plans available to you. And you can always talk to other patients in your support groups, as well as your family and friends, about which insurance plans they have found to be satisfactory.

## Insurance for Those Over Sixty-Five

1. **Medicare:** Medicare is available to citizens over age sixty-five, or those under sixty-five with a serious chronic illness, such as renal failure. Part A covers hospital charges, and Part B covers physician charges.

   What are the advantages to Medicare? It pays 80 percent of approved charges, which are nationally standardized rates that are discounted from physicians' and hospitals' usual retail charges. You can go to nearly any physician you choose, and you can always get a second opinion from any doctor that you wish, anytime, and even get third or fourth or more opinions without limit. You can get any medically necessary test any time, without preauthorization. Under regulations passed during the Clinton administration, you also can enter any approved clinical trial research study. This provision is extended by the Patient Protection and Affordable Care Act.

   If you travel, your Medicare insurance is good anywhere in the United States, but if you travel outside the country you must purchase short-term health insurance (a travel agent can identify short-term policies for you). If you have purchased a supplemental policy in addition to Medicare, it may cover you outside the United States.

What are the disadvantages? A very few physicians do not take Medicare payments; you must pay them directly and then get reimbursed by Medicare. Treatments under Medicare are subject to review and possible nonpayment by the Medicare carrier (the company that reviews Medicare claims and pays Medicare bills in your state). Several drugs and procedures are not covered by Medicare, and with health-care reform, the list of uncovered services may grow with time. You are still responsible for paying 20 percent of the standard Medicare-approved rate unless you also have Medicaid or secondary supplemental insurance (more on that in the next section). Medicare has a complex drug-reimbursement plan, and it will not pay for home antibiotic therapy. There are changes every year in Medicare coverage, so you should discuss these with your physicians every six to twelve months.

2. **Medigap, or Medicare secondary (supplemental) insurance:** This insurance is paid for privately by an individual who is over sixty-five, has Medicare, and wishes to have insurance that will take care of the 20 percent co-pay that Medicare does not pay.

What are the advantages? Medicare pays 80 percent of the Medicare-approved charges, and the secondary insurance pays the other 20 percent. Some Medicare secondary insurance companies pay for drugs up to a certain dollar amount or percentage. If you have Medigap coverage, your doctor's office very often won't require you to pay the 20 percent co-pay at the time that services are delivered, and instead will bill the Medigap insurance carrier directly for the amount that Medicare did not pay.

What are the disadvantages? Some Medigap insurance carriers do not pay for drugs. And Medigap policies will not cover a test or treatment if Medicare itself did not cover the initial 80 percent of the cost. If Medicare says that a test, procedure, or treatment you received was not medically necessary, Medicare will not pay for its 80 percent, and the Medigap policy will not pay for the other 20 percent. You won't have to pay for any of these tests either, unless you have signed an advanced beneficiary notice, or ABN. Therefore at the doctor's office or lab, you may be asked to sign an ABN, which says if Medicare does not pay for a test or procedure, you will pay it yourself. Be warned, then: if you sign that ABN notice, you will have to pay for any denied services you receive.

3. **Medicare Advantage, previously called Medicare Plus Choice (Medicare Senior HMO):** If you have Medicare, you may join an HMO plan for Medicare patients. This Medicare Part C plan is called Medicare Advantage, and it replaces Medicare Parts A and B. In joining, you surrender your Medicare card to the HMO, and you receive a card indicating you will receive care only from the doctors who participate (are contracted) with the HMO. Medicare Advantage programs use either a staff model HMO (like Kaiser Permanente medical system), or an IPA (independent practice association) model HMO. (See below for more details.)

What are the advantages? Medicare Advantage programs cover 100 percent of medically necessary tests and some or all medication costs, depending upon the plan. (Many of these plans enroll you automatically in the Medicare Part D drug program, which still requires you to pay for quite a few medications—see more about this in chapter 30, "Finding Affordable Medications.") With Medicare Advantage, you can access emergency services in most hospitals and obtain urgent care from the doctors who participate with the HMO.

What are the disadvantages? In some cases you still must make a co-payment for services. The list of allowable medications is limited, and the plan may not cover very expensive or new drugs. What you will usually notice—and what may bother you—is that there are limited choices for physicians. You must use a physician who is contracted with the plan and, in the case of an IPA model HMO, the physician must be in the *local* IPA plan. Therefore, you don't have as much choice of physicians as with standard Medicare Parts A and B. In addition, not all the doctors listed under an IPA's book of contracted doctors may be available to you, since you may be enrolled in one IPA and the doctor you want to see may be contracted with a different one. Most patients find that very frustrating, and nearly impossible to figure out from the materials they receive from the insurance company. So if you wish to visit a particular doctor, hospital, or university center, call the insurance plan first. Another frustration is that these plans offer very limited second opinions and may not cover participation in clinical trials. It has been my experience that patients in Medicare Advantage programs experience frequent delays in getting therapy due to delayed or denied authorization, and they are often seen by nurse practitioners or physicians' assistants instead of physicians.

Under the law, if you have Medicare Advantage, the plan must provide you with all the benefits you would receive from standard Medicare. But I have seen many examples of reduced benefits from HMO administrators and doctors, and the plan can deny your access to a test, treatment, or specialist consultation by deeming it "not medically necessary," which is always frustrating.

4. **Medicare Plus Medicaid:** If the income and assets of a Medicare patient are low enough, the patient may be eligible for both Medicare and Medicaid.

What are the advantages? This type of combined insurance covers 100 percent of the physician's fees, and it offers a broad choice of physicians who participate in Medicare and Medicaid programs. It also covers many medications, although the list of Medicaid-approved medicines varies by state. Second opinions are easy to get, and, in general, physicians who participate in Medicare also participate in Medicare Plus Medicaid programs (even if they otherwise do not see patients with Medicaid insurance only).

What are the disadvantages? Some physicians who accept Medicare will not accept Medicare Plus Medicaid, so check with the doctor before you make an appointment. Medicaid will not pay for all drugs; it won't cover many FDA-approved drugs unless special authorization (a TAR) is obtained. Therefore, you may experience a delay in getting certain medications paid for. Generally, however, Medicare Plus Medicaid insurance offers all the advantages of a Medicare program plus a Medigap policy. Beware, however, because in some states, patients who have Medicare Plus Medicaid will be required to enroll in a Medicaid HMO in order for Medicaid to pay for any services at all. Check with your physician, social worker, or state Medicaid office to determine your options.

5. **Accountable-Care Organizations (ACOs):** Beginning in 2003 with the Medicare Modernization Act, organizations of physicians and hospitals were formed to demonstrate that they could save costs through coordination of care. These ACOs reduced costs by using strict guidelines for care and reducing hospitalizations. At the same time they maintained the quality of care by setting performance and payment goals. The results of ACOs like Kaiser Permanente and HealthCare Partners were successful enough that the 2010 Patient Protection and Affordable Care Act allowed ACOs to contract with Medicare starting in 2012. Physicians and hospitals in your community may have formed an ACO and advertised it to you. The amount and quality of care you will get through an ACO will vary. That's because care may be given one of two ways: under a capitated fee schedule (so your doctor receives the same amount for your care, regardless of whether she sees you, and regardless of the procedures or tests she does), or under the traditional fee-for-service schedule (so your doctor is paid only for each actual visit or test). Therefore, before you join an ACO, check on its reputation and the satisfaction of its patients, and find out how much care patients in the program actually receive. Because physician pay may increase or decrease depending on the internal rules of each ACO, primary-care physicians and specialists may tend to join or drop out of the ACO fairly frequently, which could lead to disruptions in your care.

## Insurance for Those Under Sixty-Five

1. **Indemnity Insurance:** Patients who have an indemnity type of insurance plan have the broadest range of access to health care.

What are the advantages? You have free choice of nearly any physician, with insurance typically covering 80 percent of the physician's usual and customary charges, while you pay the other 20 percent. Indemnity insurance may cover research trials, and it is accepted nearly anywhere in the United States and, with some plans, even in foreign countries. (Check these provisions in various policies before you purchase one.) Many indemnity policies also cover medications, with a co-payment.

The disadvantages of indemnity programs are that they are very expensive, and their premiums may jump annually. Nevertheless, many companies still provide indemnity insurance plans for their employees at a discount, or for free. If you're considering indemnity insurance, compare its rates with those of the other plans listed below.

2. **Preferred Provider Organizations (PPOs):** PPO insurance is similar to indemnity insurance, but you are given a discounted rate if you use physicians who are contracted with the PPO. Under that contract, the physician agrees to accept a reduced rate from the PPO in exchange for being recommended to all the PPO's beneficiaries. A PPO typically pays 70 to 80 percent of the discounted rate after the annual deductible amount has been met; you pay the remainder.

   The advantages of a PPO are that you have a free choice of any physician within the plan at a discounted rate, but you can also receive care from physicians outside the plan. Keep in mind, however, that if you go outside the contracted physician network, you will be responsible for all charges in excess of the rate that a PPO-contracted doctor would receive. This can be a considerable amount—you may end up paying 50 to 70 percent of the charges of the non-contracted doctor.

   The disadvantages are that with a PPO, the "utilization review"—that is, the process of determining which requested services will be covered or denied—is slightly more restrictive than with an indemnity plan, although it is much *less* restrictive than with an HMO. Utilization review might, therefore, deem some services "not medically indicated" and refuse to authorize them for you. PPOs require prior authorization for certain services (the PPO contract will list them). And although a PPO is less expensive than an indemnity plan, it is more expensive than an HMO, and the premium may also increase annually.

Some employers do not offer PPO insurance to employees. If you want a PPO plan but your company doesn't offer one, contact the human-resources office at work or an insurance agent to find out if there's a way you can get a PPO-type plan offered, even if you have to pay extra for it, or if your employer can apply its HMO contribution toward PPO plans. Some employers will offer a higher salary to employees who do not take the company's health insurance, allowing them to shop for their own personal plan outside of work. You can get more information from your company's human-resources office.

3. **HMO Staff Model Insurance:** An example of this type of insurance is the Kaiser Permanente medical system. The staff model HMO hires its own medical staff or contracts with a medical staff (in the case of Kaiser, it is Permanente Medical Group). The medical group is a closed panel; you cannot go outside the Kaiser system to obtain other care unless you pay for all the services yourself. The only exceptions are certain highly specialized services, which are provided by outside doctors or institutions under contract with Kaiser (for example, heart or bone marrow transplants sometimes are obtained outside the Kaiser system).

There are several advantages of the HMO staff model. First, this type of plan is usually (but not always) cheaper than a PPO. There is no, or a very low, co-payment required from you. In some cases, you may have access to research clinical trials. The HMO staff model covers many medications, although some expensive or new drugs may not be provided without special approval. Because patients always see the same staff, these plans foster considerable patient loyalty. Generally, patients who are not very sick evaluate this sort of plan quite favorably; patients who are very sick tend to give it a far poorer approval rating. (This usually varies, depending on the nature of the illness.)

The disadvantages? You have a very limited choice of physicians (and in many cases, you actually see a nurse practitioner or physician's assistant instead). You may experience considerable delays until certain treatments are authorized, and if you are very sick, you might become frustrated because a treatment you have heard about in the newspaper or in patient support groups isn't available to you. Many treatments commonly covered in PPO plans may not be authorized by this type of insurance.

4. **The HMO IPA (Independent Practice Association) Model:** Under this type of plan, you are assigned to a particular IPA in one section of a city, and the doctors contracted with that particular IPA are the only doctors to whom you have access. For example, if you live in the East San Gabriel Valley of Los Angeles, you would be assigned to an IPA in the East San Gabriel Valley. A doctor in west Los Angeles might be contracted by the same HMO but affiliated with a different local IPA, so he would not be available to you.

The main advantage of the IPA model HMO is that it is usually cheaper than all other insurance programs. It typically pays for at least some medications, but only up to a specified amount, and usually for only a very limited list of drugs. This program rarely allows you to participate in clinical trials, but occasionally it will make an exception with special authorization.

The disadvantages are that this plan offers a very limited choice of providers, and there can be considerable delays until the utilization review committee authorizes a special treatment you may feel is required. With this HMO model also, you often see nurse practitioners and physicians' assistants for primary-care physician visits.

If you have an HMO plan, it is important to find out which doctors in the plan deliver very high-quality medicine. (Practically every HMO plan has many of these doctors.) You must ask many questions and get plenty of advice, as explained in chapter 1, so that your care is comprehensive, efficient, and excellent.

5. **The HMO with Point-of-Service (POS) Option:** With this plan, you have an IPA model HMO, but you may elect to see a physician outside the HMO (the point of service). In that circumstance, the HMO will pay a limited part of the doctor's bill.

The advantages are that you can go outside the HMO and get care from any other doctor. You can get second opinions and lifesaving therapy, even if the HMO refuses to authorize such treatment for you.

The disadvantages are that the HMO with POS option costs more than an HMO itself, and it typically pays only 30 to 60 percent of the services of a non-IPA physician.

6. **Medicaid:** If you have limited resources, you may be eligible for the Medicaid program. This program is administered by each state, and the state determines its own eligibility criteria. Eligibility, therefore, varies from state to state. If participating in a Medicaid program, you may be assigned to an HMO, which would have the same disadvantages as the IPA or staff model HMOs listed above.

The advantages of Medicaid are that many drugs are routinely available to you (although the Medicaid list of approved medications is somewhat limited), and that you may go to any physician who accepts Medicaid payments.

The disadvantages are that many physicians do not accept Medicaid, and this often limits the accessibility of doctors you need. Due to the eligibility restrictions of many Medicaid programs, some patients may be required to pay a "share of costs" that can be hundreds of dollars a month.

7. **Health Savings Account (HSA):** Created in 2003 by the Medicare Modernization Act, and modified in 2010 by the Patient Protection and Affordable Care Act, the HSA is becoming a more popular option for paying for medical services. Many businesses now provide an HSA together with a high-deductible health plan (HDHP) instead of standard

PPO or HMO insurance. Consider this option, even if you think you have a good HDHP plan already—it may have particular advantages for younger and healthier individuals. Before you decide that this is the best method of obtaining medical care, however, discuss it with a good health-insurance agent—or better yet, two or three.

With an HSA, you pay money into a savings account each month, just as you would pay monthly health-insurance premiums. The savings account pays for two things: qualified medical expenses (e.g., doctor, dentist, vision, counseling, chiropractor, physical therapy), and prescription medications before you have met your HDHP deductible amount (usually $2,000 to $5,000 annually). Maximum HSA contributions in 2012 are $3,100 for individuals and $6,250 for families.

If you do not require any medical care during the year, or if you require medical care costing less than the amount in your savings account, the excess money in the account is accumulated (rolled over) for future years. Later, the savings account can be used to purchase other health-care insurance (Medicare supplemental insurance or long-term care policies, for example). If you do not spend what you've saved in the HSA, it can be rolled into an IRA-like plan and then used for any expenses after retirement. Check out the details of any plan you're considering with an insurance agent or your employer's human-resources department. (Since HSAs are available to any employer, a self-employed individual can choose this plan, as well.)

Among the advantages of HSAs are that the payments are tax-free and can be applied to a wide variety of medical expenses, and they save on FICA and Medicare taxes as well. Younger and healthier people tend to like this option, but older individuals do not. A big disadvantage is that in order to save money, people with HSAs and HDHPs tend to delay necessary health care and physician appointments and skip medications.

Another type of plan is the **Flexible Spending Account**, which is also tax-free and is available only through a cafeteria plan set up by an employer. The maximum annual contribution is $2,500. Although it can be used for any eligible medical care, including over-the-counter drugs, this is a use-it-by-end-of-the-year-or-lose-it program—funds not paid out toward medical expenses are forfeited at end of year.

Although an HSA account is owned by the individual, another plan, the **Health Reimbursement Arrangement**, is owned by the employer. It can cover eligible medical expenses, it does not need to be used with any other health plan (like the HDHP), and any unused funds roll over to future years. This plan must be set up by the employer.

8. **Hospital-Only Insurance:** If regular insurance, which covers both physicians and hospitals, is still too expensive for you, there are plans that cover only hospitals. These plans (sometimes called "savers") require evidence of insurability, and are based on PPO models, which require you to use only contracted hospitals. These plans have varying deductibles (the amount you have to pay before the insurance begins to cover your hospital care). The total deductible to be paid before there is 100 percent coverage of all remaining charges can vary from policy to policy as well. Still, if you can't afford another, more expensive plan, a hospital-only program may offer you a way to avoid catastrophic health-care bills for sudden injury or illness. The disadvantage is that outpatient doctor fees, laboratory tests, medications, and X-rays are not covered or discounted, so you still have to pay for all of them. To find out about this type of insurance, you must contact an insurance agent.

## Impact of the Affordable Care Act

The Patient Protection and Affordable Care Act ("ObamaCare") has many provisions helpful to people. In addition to requiring private insurance plans to cover prevention and screening for illnesses (see chapter 9), and mandating that private plans cover patient-care costs in certain research clinical trials (see chapter 17), the act allows children to stay on their parents' health plans until age twenty-six. Also, there are no caps on lifetime payments by the insurance company, helping patients with expensive life-threatening illnesses such as cardiovascular disease or cancer. Most importantly, the act prevents insurance plans from denying coverage to people based on preexisting conditions. For people whose employers do not provide health insurance, many states will have insurance exchanges through which people can find more affordable medical insurance. If this act is changed by new regulations, or is amended (or repealed), these provisions may change. You can obtain more information from your doctor, employer, insurance agent, or health plan if you hear about changes occurring.

## Sources of Insurance Benefits

If you are younger than sixty-five and employed, your employer is likely the source of your health insurance. Large companies often provide a choice of several different types of health insurance, each with a different cost. Once you've been presented with those choices, you should carefully evaluate each plan and its benefits, exclusions, and costs. If you are confused, ask the person responsible for the insurance benefits (often the director of the human-resources department) about the exact nature of each option. (Is it an HMO, HMO with POS option, or PPO?) Only after understanding the characteristics of each plan should you decide which one is best for you.

Take this decision very seriously; read all the coverage terms and think about them. My patient Darcy, for example, was offered a choice of health plans when she started working for a large company. She was happy to have the choice, but she leaned toward the least expensive option because she wanted to save money to buy a stereo system. "What, are you crazy?" asked her sister Ann. "Look at this HMO policy you want to pick. You can't even go to our community hospital! And if you were to get cancer, this exclusion says you can't get chemotherapy unless you buy the expensive rider to pay for it."

Because their mom had developed breast cancer five years before and needed chemotherapy to cure her, Darcy listened to Ann's advice and chose the more expensive PPO plan without the exclusions and restrictions. Two months later, Darcy found a lump in her breast. After cancer was diagnosed, she needed $50,000 of chemotherapy treatments to cure her illness, just as her mom had. As Darcy said later, "You never know when you'll need to use the insurance, so better get the best up-front."

If you are unemployed, self-employed, or employed by a company not offering health insurance, look into organizations from which you can obtain group health insurance. For example, are you eligible for group insurance as part of a club, union, church group, chamber of commerce, fraternity, or sorority? You should check with a health-insurance agent about group plan eligibility.

As a result of health-care reform legislation in many states, as well as the 2010 Patient Protection and Affordable Care Act, by 2014 all states may establish health-insurance exchanges to provide insurance choices for low-income individuals not eligible for Medicaid, and otherwise uninsurable patients. The cost of these insurance policies is still unknown, but it will be subsidized for low-income individuals. Until 2014, a national high-risk insurance pool will be available for those who cannot find insurance (usually due to preexisting conditions). Therefore, it is important to determine your eligibility by checking with state insurance offices through NCSL.org/?tabid=14329 and with the federal government health exchange through HealthCare.gov. Also, be aware that children can now remain on their parents' health-insurance policies until age twenty-six.

Under provisions of the Patient Protection and Affordable Care Act, by 2014 qualified health plans must provide certain common benefits, setting a standard across all plans. Because of this, health-insurance programs will tend to be more similar—and more expensive.

## Long-Term Care Insurance and Nursing Facilities

As the American life expectancy continues to increase, it becomes more likely that you will need skilled nursing-facility care, home-nursing support, or long-term nursing-home care for a chronic condition (e.g., Alzheimer's disease, stroke, emphysema, heart failure, or spinal disease). In 1986, only 29 percent of people who died after age twenty-five used nursing-home care at some point in their lives. It's anticipated that by 2020, 46 percent of people over age sixty-five will at some point be in a nursing home. Among those using nursing homes, 55 percent use them for at least one year, and 21 percent use them for more than five years. Some 25 percent of women and 15 percent of men live in nursing homes for more than five years.

So how will you pay for extraordinarily expensive nursing-home care for you or your spouse? At present, this is not a problem for those with Medicaid, which covers skilled nursing-facility care and long-term nursing-home charges. If you have Medicare insurance and you qualify for skilled nursing-facility care, your charges for that care will be fully covered for the first twenty days, only partially covered for days twenty-one through one hundred, and not covered at all after one hundred days. PPO insurance coverage varies, but it has limitations similar to those of Medicare.

If you want to ensure that you can afford the care that will protect your health and quality of life, I highly recommend buying long-term care insurance. Shopping for that insurance can be confusing, however, so make sure you do your research. In addition to using a health-care insurance agent (whose advice is free, but who will really want you to purchase the insurance he represents), you can get good information online at NAIC. org/documents/consumer_alert_ltc.pdf and Long-Term-Care-Insurance-Planners.com.

If you have PPO, HMO, or ACO insurance, check with your agent or your employer's human-resources department for details on your current coverage for skilled nursing care. Make sure that you are prepared for the eventuality of short- or long-term nursing-home needs. In the process, you'll avoid the possibility of overwhelming personal expense and even bankruptcy.

Once you know you have coverage for nursing-facility care (or you have arranged to pay for it yourself), how do you choose the best facility? After considering the advice of your physician, nurses, and hospital discharge planner, check out the nursing-home ratings and recommendations at Medicare.gov/nhcompare. Then visit nursing facilities to check out their staff, cleanliness, smell, appearance, and services/activities.

### Communicating with Your Insurance Company

Once you have procured health insurance, keep a list of your insurance company contacts: the information center, benefits and coverage office, authorizations or utilization review office, appeals office, patient advocacy or complaints office, and medical director's office. And always keep a record of every call you make to your insurance company, noting with whom you spoke, when, and what was said. Different individuals at an insurance company can give you slightly different answers to your questions, so knowing who told you what and when can make appealing a denial or other potentially detrimental decision easier and more successful.

## Tips

- Know about every type of insurance available to you.
- Reevaluate your insurance choice annually.
- Never go uninsured.
- Know with whom you can talk (and complain, if necessary) at the insurance company.

## Contemporary Medicine and Medical Insurance

Health-care reform concentrates on several issues, and among the most important is the health-insurance system. The above discussion includes numerous examples of state and national reforms to insurance that are in the process of being implemented.

It's safe to say that the process of reforming insurance will never end. The number of laws and regulations enacted over the last two decades alone suggest that the rate of change will only increase. Of course, this is a direct effect of public outrage over rising insurance costs and the care of uninsured patients. And while modern medicine offers ever newer and better services—like robotic surgery, advanced radiologic scanning, cutting-edge medications, and better cardiac catheters—employers and patients have been adversely affected by the increased insurance costs required to pay for these advanced services.

Since you can expect changes in insurance every few months, you should know how to access the resources that will tell you if there have been changes in your benefits, or that will help you decide if you should modify your health-care plan during the annual window when you can choose different insurance. If you are over sixty-five, you should rely on the Department of Health and Human-Resources website, HHS.gov, to learn about annual changes to insurance and to locate a health-care insurance agent who can offer guidance. If you are under sixty-five, consult a health-care insurance agent and your employer's human-resources department. If you are financially challenged, use the resources of your state health department and contact a social worker at a community health center or hospital to help you identify your best options.

# Chapter 26

# Understanding Your Insurance Bill and EOB

## Health Care Costs and Bills

Bills you receive from physicians, clinics, and hospitals are always expensive. And even worse, these bills are complex—sometimes nearly incomprehensible. Fortunately, every office and hospital has a billing expert who can help you understand each charge. Whenever you receive a medical bill, carefully examine it to be certain that you understand each charge and that no erroneous items have been added, as errors are very common. The billing expert can go over your record with you to verify each charge.

After receiving any service from a doctor or hospital, the first paper you will receive is the bill from the provider of the service (not from your insurance). Usually, your insurance will pay part of the bill for each service you received, so don't pay the first bill you get from the doctor or hospital; it was sent to let you know what charges will be sent to your insurance company. However, when you open that first bill, you should review each item on it to be certain that you actually received the service. If you are at all confused, call the billing expert at the doctor's office or hospital (or whoever sent you the bill) and ask her to walk you through the charges for verification. She will also confirm that the initial bill does not have to be paid and will be submitted directly to your insurance company.

If there is a mistake on your bill, ask the billing expert at the doctor's office or hospital to mail you a written correction. Keep a record of the person with whom you spoke, the date and time, and the action that was promised. Then immediately notify your insurance company that the bill will be corrected by the provider.

The second paper you will receive is an explanation of benefits (EOB) from your insurance company. This is not a bill, so again, do not pay anything yet. The EOB will give you the following information:

1.  The provider of the service (the hospital, doctor, lab, etc.).
2.  The date of the service.
3.  The retail charge (the amount you saw on the first bill).
4.  The amount that is allowed or covered (the discounted charge arranged by the insurance company on your behalf).
5.  The amount that your insurance company will pay. (If you have already met your deductible for the year, this is usually 80 percent of the allowed charge, but it can vary depending on your health plan.) Remember that until you have paid the total deductible, the insurance company may not pay anything, but you still will only have to pay the discounted price, not the full retail price (your insurance has already helped you).
6.  The amount that you must pay the doctor, hospital, etc. (This includes the amounts for your deductible and co-pay.)

Since the EOB is not a bill, merely an explanation, you should not pay anything after receiving it. However, if there has been any correction of the original charges from the doctor or hospital, make sure the charges have been corrected in the charges column of the EOB. If they haven't, notify the insurance company and request a revised EOB. If you have any questions about the amounts charged to you or about charges not covered by insurance, call the billing office whose phone number is listed on the EOB. As before, keep a record of the phone call; write a note on the EOB itself or on a separate sheet of paper you staple to the EOB.

Sometimes you'll receive an EOB that says you owe 100 percent of the charge from a laboratory or imaging center with no payment or adjustment from the insurance company. This is a common error; often it happens when the laboratory or imaging center sends insurance, Medicare, or Medicaid an incomplete bill (usually missing your correct diagnosis, insurance number, or date of birth). Perhaps your doctor didn't send the diagnosis to the lab or radiology center, or maybe it wasn't the right diagnosis for the test. If this happens to you, call the billing office at the laboratory or imaging center. If they need a "covered" diagnosis which will be paid by insurance, call the doctor's office and ask that a clerk, medical assistant, or nurse send the corrected diagnosis to the laboratory or radiology center so it can resubmit the bill to insurance. Insist that they do this rapidly so that interest charges don't start building up. (That said, interest charges can always be voided, so don't let the lab or imaging center charge you any interest if your insurance agrees to cover the bill.)

The last paper you will receive will be a bill from the doctor's office, hospital laboratory, imaging center, or other health-service provider. This lists the final amount for you to pay. Check this amount against the amount the EOB says you owe. If the numbers agree, it is time to take out your checkbook or credit card and pay the bill.

Remember, if you still have questions, do not pay until they have all been answered, not matter how long it takes. But keep in touch with the billing director or supervisor, and keep records of all your calls or letters to reconcile any disagreements. These errors and disagreements are very common, so do not be embarrassed about contacting the office, hospital, or insurance company. For example, you may have been instructed to pay an amount that has not been discounted; you may have been instructed to pay before the insurance payment was credited to the account or before your secondary insurance (if you have any) was credited to the account; or the office may have billed you for a service despite being told by insurance that it was not supposed to (because the service was already bundled into another charge).

After you have met your annual deductible payment, and if you have both primary and secondary insurance, be especially suspicious of any charge remaining to be paid, since the combination usually covers absolutely all services. And if you have a PPO or Medicare without supplemental insurance, check for problems if you've been asked to pay more than 20 percent of any allowed charge in the EOB.

## Tips

- Know the difference between an EOB and a bill.
- Only pay a bill if it seems correct. Never pay an incorrect bill or remit payment based solely on the EOB.
- If you have questions about the EOB or the bill, call the insurance company and call your doctor … and keep detailed notes.

## Today's Medicine and Bills

One of the concerns addressed by health-care reforms is patients' difficulty with forms, bills, EOBs, and insurance companies' communication with patients. Unfortunately, the insurance industry's attempts to make it all clearer have resulted in even longer forms and more confusion for a lot of patients. So don't feel alone if you are frustrated or baffled by your medical bills. The answers are just a few e-mails or phone calls away: to your doctor's billing clerk or supervisor, and to your insurance agent. So if the insurance company is giving you grief, check the recommendations above—and don't give up.

As more health-care reforms are implemented, it becomes more likely that you'll want to or have to change your insurance. Your new plan might have different coverage, and its EOBs may look less familiar. Even your physician's office may have a little trouble billing correctly with a new insurance plan. So do expect some problems along the journey to newer and (we hope) better health care.

# Chapter 27

# Health-Insurance Problems

## Typical Insurance Plan Problems

There are common problems that go along with insurance coverage. You likely will be angry and frustrated if you encounter one of these issues:

- **Your insurance fails to cover common services such as health screenings or preventive care.** If there are services you wish to have covered, carefully compare insurance plans before you buy one to be certain that coverage is provided and the specific services important to you are not excluded. (Sometimes common services are so cheap, however, that you'll find it more economical to pay for such services privately, out of pocket, rather than choosing a very expensive plan that covers them.)
- **Your insurance plan fails to authorize coverage of medically needed services, despite your physician's requests for that authorization.** Before you choose your health plan, ask your physician's office staff whether it has problems with the specific insurance plan you are considering, and if so, how often.
- **Your doctor or hospital is not contracted with your new insurance plan.** Before purchasing an insurance plan, call your physicians and hospital to be certain they are on the plan.

If they are not, the offices usually can suggest insurance plans that would cover their services.

- **You erroneously use a doctor or hospital not contracted with your insurance.** Before using any doctor, hospital, laboratory, radiology center, or health-care supplier, always ask if it is contracted with your insurance, and then confirm that with a call to the insurance company. Although you may have a booklet listing all contracted physicians and hospitals, it is wise to confirm the information with the billing office; insurance contracts may expire before a new provider book is sent out, so you may actually be relying on an outdated list. You should keep a record of any confirmation of coverage by a medical office or your insurance company.

- **Your insurance plan has a very low maximum payment for certain services or a low total dollar limit for all benefits.** Beware of cheap insurance plans that provide a very small amount of coverage or a very limited maximum payment. Carefully compare plans, noting the benefit limits, before purchasing one. If you need help determining what those limits are, call the billing expert in your doctor's office or hospital, or an insurance agent.

- **Your insurance company denies payment for services because your doctor has not given the appropriate diagnosis.** For example, you have anemia and your doctor ordered a blood test for your vitamin B12 level, but the doctor's office did not note the anemia diagnosis in the lab request. The insurance company denies payment because it does not know you have anemia, so the lab bills you for the test. If you get billed for a test that is not covered, ask the insurance company exactly why they did not pay, and then call the doctor's office and ask them to submit the necessary diagnosis to the lab, hospital, or radiology center that provided the service. Do not pay the bill yourself when this type of error occurs.

## Termination of Employment

If you are insured through you employer and you resign or are terminated from your job, you face a health-insurance crisis. Most people in this situation consider using COBRA (Consolidated Omnibus Budget Reconciliation Act, a 1986 federal law), the federally mandated protection for employees of companies with a staff of twenty or more. COBRA allows you to leave a company but keep your health insurance for another eighteen months (or thirty-six months, if you lose employer-paid insurance due to divorce or death). You do have to pay for the insurance—and usually it is expensive—but coverage is continuous for that designated period until you get another job with insurance or until you have located another insurance plan.

It is most important to have *no lapse* in insurance, because many health plans will reduce your coverage or benefits due to risks or preexisting conditions once your original plan has lapsed. Before you leave a job, therefore, contact the human-resources office or an insurance agent so you are aware of all possible options for continuing your coverage.

For those whose COBRA eligibility has expired, each state is required to have other insurance available, regardless of preexisting conditions, under federal HIPAA regulations (Health Insurance Portability and Accountability Act of 1996). Contact your state insurance commissioner for information about available plans (see appendix 4).

## Preexisting Conditions

If you are about to begin a new insurance plan, you will be asked about all your prior illnesses. If you have had a disease or condition, or if you have active symptoms, you may be declined insurance because of preexisting illness (or you may have to pay a higher premium). What can you do about this? If the prior illness has disappeared, get a letter from the physicians who treated you stating that the illness is no longer present and that there is no risk of recurrence. You can also check with other health plans to see if they will insure you without a preexisting condition, since criteria for what constitutes a preexisting condition varies among health-insurance companies.

If an insurance company wants to issue a policy excluding a preexisting disease from coverage, find out if a major medical policy can be written without the exclusion. Also, you may be able to join a large group or go to work for a larger employer whose health insurance has no preexisting exclusions. Check with an insurance agent to learn about all your options.

As I've noted, there is a national high-risk insurance pool for individuals who have been uninsured for six months due to a preexisting condition; several states have their own high-risk pools as well. And in 2014, if current legislation is not amended or repealed, all insurance programs may have to accept individuals regardless of preexisting conditions. These high-risk plans may be expensive, but having health insurance is critical, especially if you have a preexisting condition.

## Discussing Rates with Your Physician

If you are paying your physician (and nearly every patient outside of an HMO or Medicaid program must at least make co-payments for many services), you may feel that the costs are too high for you to afford. Is there any way to get a reduction in rates?

You can almost always discuss rates with your doctor's office manager or with the hospital, and in some instances you can get a discount on your bill or arrange to pay it on an installment plan. Why? Despite many people's impression that physicians and hospitals are anxious to charge patients as much as they can, many medical providers are very compassionate, and they may offer you a discount if you truly are having trouble paying their usual charges. If you hope to negotiate lower fees or arrange an installment plan, however, it's best to have such discussions before you've used the provider's services.

One possibility is asking for a discount if you pay cash in advance, either for the total charge or for the co-payment. And in rare instances, a medical provider will accept the insurance payment alone as payment in full for a particular service, so it never hurts to ask if this is possible if you would otherwise be forced to use a different doctor or hospital. If you have a whole-life insurance policy, check with the life-insurance carrier to see if you can borrow money from your equity (cash value) in the policy to pay your medical bills.

Before you try to negotiate a discount with a medical provider, go to the website of the American Medical Association to see what Medicare pays doctors for a particular service. Visit AMA.org/cpt, and you'll see all the services a physician may provide, listed by CPT code. Once you know the rates Medicare pays, you'll have an idea of how much of a discount the physician's office might be willing to provide (since many doctors' offices accept Medicare rates). If you are embarrassed about discussing this with the office manager or physician, ask a family member, a friend, or even a lawyer to make the call for you.

If you are expecting high physician bills that you won't be able to pay, consider having a negotiator service call the physician's office to work out a manageable solution. You can find information about negotiator services online at ProtectiveSmartHealthPremier.com or UninsuredBillReview.com.

## Tips

- Problems will always exist with health insurance companies, because they are trying to save money. Expect to have to deal with them.
- Rely on your doctor's office staff for help with insurance problems.
- Find an experienced insurance broker who can guide you through the problems.

## Today's Medicine and Insurance Problems

Much of health-care reform has been aimed at the insurance industry, but as with any change, implementing those reforms has come with a lot of problems. New types of insurance policies will create new problems. New benefits will mean new regulations. New types of treatments will require new eligibility rules. I anticipate even more problems as we advance, so keeping your health-care team together and on your side will be ever more important.

# Chapter 28

# Insurance Company Authorizations for Your Care

One of the most challenging aspects of medical care is requesting, waiting for, and then getting (or being denied) authorization for tests or treatments. There are several approaches you can take to deal with these frustrations.

If your insurance company has an authorization process (and almost all of them do), its approval or denial of a request for your care often depends upon *how that request is made*. Actually, insurance plans do approve most requests for authorization, and needed care is appropriately given. Once your doctor requests an authorization, a clerk or nurse at the insurance company compares that request to a set of standard authorized treatments. If the treatment *as requested* is on the list approved for the diagnosis *as described by the doctor*, then it is authorized. Only in rare circumstances does a physician perform the initial review; most insurance plans use clerks or nurses.

Unfortunately, clerks, nurses, and medical directors sometimes make mistakes. When that happens, your insurance may fail to authorize medically necessary treatments that might benefit you. As a result of their decision, your condition may worsen, you may experience more and needless suffering, and you might even die. At the very least, such a denial causes great anxiety and anger. When appealing the denial of a treatment I felt was medically necessary for a patient, I have actually been told by an insurance company, "Just because we deny authorization doesn't mean you can't still treat the patient with the procedure. You'll just have to have the patient pay for it himself." The fact is, most procedures and treatments are too costly for patients to afford without insurance reimbursement. More important, by paying your insurance premiums, you have already paid to receive necessary and appropriate care.

Patients and doctors alike often feel that many insurance denials are self-serving. After all, the more denials or delays in authorization for tests or treatments, the higher the profit for the insurance company.

But sometimes a denial occurs because the requesting doctor's office left out critical information when they asked for treatment authorization. It can be a clerical omission, like submitting the wrong birth date or health plan identification number, or the office might not have submitted the right diagnosis or accurately described the procedure in question. And sometimes the denial is just an incorrect decision by the insurance company.

Tragically, insurance denials can result in considerable suffering. My patient June had metastatic melanoma, a very aggressive skin cancer that had spread to her leg and lymph nodes. She was in complete remission from chemotherapy when her husband's employer changed their insurance to an HMO, and June had to see other doctors. After other doctors stopped her chemotherapy, her melanoma returned and she developed a knee infection. The HMO delayed approval for knee surgery to cure the infection and denied her appeals for further treatments and chemotherapy. Ultimately, this resulted in amputation of her leg and recurrence of her melanoma. I was surprised to see June return to my office a few months later. "Well, Dr. Presant, I'm finally back here with you again," she said. "You can't believe what I had to go through to get approved to be here. My husband Jack deserves all the credit. He wrote letters to the state health commissioner, and then he called this nice lady in the commissioner's office. That lady called the HMO, and suddenly I got this approval letter saying I could see you and get the same chemotherapy again. It seems like magic … I guess the system works once in a while." June restarted her chemotherapy treatments, and the cancer disappeared, just as it had before. Now, years later, June remains in complete remission.

## What Should You Expect from Your Insurance Company and Your Physician?

- If you require a test or a treatment that necessitates authorization, you should expect the authorization process to be **timely**. If it is an emergency, you should be able to obtain authorization within the day; if it is urgent, within the week. If an authorization is delayed, ask your doctor's staff to call immediately to speed up the process. At the same time, call your insurance company to ask the medical director or his staff to facilitate the processing of the request. Follow up this request with a letter.

- You should expect the authorization request from the physician's office to be **accurate**. The diagnosis should be correct, the description of the symptoms should be appropriate, the request should be immediate, and the documentation provided should be sufficient to support the request. If necessary, the physician's office should also supply copies of medical reports confirming the effectiveness of the proposed treatment or surgery.

- You should expect the authorization or denial to be **appropriate** to your illness and condition. If there is a denial of authorization, it should be in writing with the reasons given, and you and your doctor should be given the name of the responsible reviewer or medical director.

- You should expect your appeal of a denial to get a **prompt** decision, with review by appropriate medical specialists who are familiar with your type of illness. After any denial, the insurance company should immediately provide a written description of the appeal process, so that you and your physician can begin the appeal as soon as possible.

As soon as you receive a denial, have your physician appeal the denial using the insurance company's regular process. If you need the test or treatment urgently, ask your physician if he could also call the insurance plan's medical director to emphasize the need for immediate approval.

When you appeal a denial to the insurance company, you may want to use the sample letter I have written for you (see appendix 5). Make sure to send a copy to the state insurance commissioner as well.

The results of appeals at two HMO organizations were reviewed by Harvard University and RAND Corporation researchers, who published their findings in the February 19, 2003, issue of the *Journal of the American Medical Association.* After studying more than seventeen hundred appeals, the authors found that patients won more than half the appeals about the medical necessity of a treatment, but only about one-third of appeals about using an out-of-network physician or about contractual coverage (when, for example, a test was medically necessary but not covered by the insurance contract). When you and your doctor fight together, the insurance company will often relent.

If your insurance company continues to deny a request for tests or treatment, consider the following solutions:

- Personally and promptly **appeal the decision in writing** to the utilization review committee (or the individual responsible for utilization review), sending copies to the president of the insurance company and the state insurance commissioner, stating why you expect approval—for example, "I expected this request to be approved because it was medically indicated and recommended by my physician, who is a specialist in my illness." Both you and your physician should appeal the denial individually.
- **Consider obtaining a second opinion** from another physician to confirm the medical necessity of the procedure. This worked for a fifty-six-year-old patient of mine with lung cancer. I needed additional information about the extent of the disease in order to plan an appropriate treatment, so I requested a PET scan (an expensive test that can detect otherwise hidden lung cancer metastases in other organs). My request was denied, as was my appeal. So the patient obtained a second opinion from another physician who confirmed the necessity for the PET scan, which was then approved. See chapter 25 on choosing your health insurance and chapter 15 for advice on getting a second opinion from an HMO.
- **Have the physician's office submit an appeal with additional data.** For example, the doctor might include a more complete description of your symptoms and the necessity for prompt action, or she might submit a recent medical article indicating

the usefulness of the requested treatment. Urge your physician's office to explain specifically why your particular diagnosis and the severity of your condition require prompt authorization and justify a particular test or treatment. (If a test has been requested, remind the doctor to indicate to the insurance company that this is *not* a screening test, as such tests often are not covered by insurance.)

- If you still do not get approval for a needed treatment, **consider having a lawyer write a letter** (on legal letterhead, of course) to the insurance company and the state insurance commissioner demanding prompt authorization for the requested treatments, which are medically necessary. In my experience, even if a physician and patient have written strong letters, many insurance companies respond more promptly and favorably to a lawyer's letter.

- If you and your physician feel the treatment is a necessity even though the insurance company has denied it, discuss with your doctor whether you should just **pay for the treatment yourself**. This will allow you to get the appropriate treatment promptly so your illness does not get worse. After the treatment has begun, you can consider suing the insurance company to pay for the test or treatment your physician felt was *medically necessary* to care for your condition.

- If your insurance company denied authorization for a medically necessary test or treatment and you ended up paying for it yourself, you can opt to **sue the insurance company in small claims court** (if your state has one). Surprisingly, this option was originally suggested to me by the medical director of an insurance company. You do not need an attorney to sue in small claims court. If you are considering a suit, you should have your doctor's letter stating your diagnosis, the test or treatment requested, and the medical necessity of that test or treatment in your case. You should also have the written letter of denial from the insurance company along with documentation showing that you appealed the decision promptly and that even the appeal was denied. I have been told that in cases where all such documentation is submitted, the judge usually rules in favor of the patient. Sometimes, just the threat of suit convinces an insurance company to approve a request.

- **Use the state insurance commissioner** to review your denial and possibly intercede on your behalf. In fighting her melanoma, my patient June was refused authorization to continue her ongoing care with me because I was not contracted with the new health plan her employer required her to use. After her husband contacted the state department of insurance, which intervened on her behalf, the insurance company promptly reversed its decision and authorized the continuing treatments.

As a patient, is this too difficult for you to even consider—to fight for the tests and treatments that can save your life, reduce your suffering, or lengthen your survival? With endlessly tightening restrictions on insurance payments, sometimes you just have to be strong and take action yourself to get what you need. And you will feel that you have really accomplished a lot when you get that approval. Unfortunately, I have had patients who were unwilling to confront the insurance company—who just shrugged their shoulders, saying, "Well, just do what they'll pay for." If the doctor is willing to give you the information you need, you and your family should have the tenacity and joint courage to make the phone calls and write the letters necessary to get the best care you can. The best news is, most insurance companies ultimately want to do the right thing for the patient. By asking appropriately and repeatedly (if necessary), and by working with your physician, you can almost always obtain the treatments you need.

## Tips

- Expect occasional denials of requested tests or treatments.
- Work with the billing personnel at the doctor's office to initiate the appeal.
- Expect a prompt and accurate decision on the appeal.
- Use other resources (an insurance agent, the state health commissioner, or even a lawyer) to get the care you need promptly so that you do not suffer.

## Modern Medicine and Insurance Denials

Constantly evolving changes in insurance programs and authorizations are a universal corollary of health-care reforms, whether legislated or insurance-market driven. In order for insurers and the government to reduce health-care costs, you must expect these changes to affect the approvals process for your care. Denials will probably increase, appeals will become more necessary, and this administrative process will become more frustrating.

By staying calm and acting promptly—using your physician, second opinions, your state insurance commissioner, and a lawyer, if necessary— you should be able to get the care you need. But you can also minimize your risk of inappropriate denials by carefully shopping for your insurance and purchasing from a reputable company. (Check out the Internet to see other patients' experiences with the insurance company you're considering.) And always maintaining your insurance will avoid the frustration of experiencing denials based on a preexisting condition.

# Chapter 29

# The Financially Poor and the Medically Poor

First, consider the tragic example of my patient Mrs. Jones. "I had no insurance, no money, nothing to pay for a doctor's visit!" she told me. "Where was I to go?" I met Mrs. Jones in the hospital, where I was seeing her in consultation for a lump in her breast. She lived alone, and she had very little money and no family. Although she could feel the lump in her breast, she had no physician, and so she didn't do anything—she just disregarded the mass. When I saw her, unfortunately, the results showed a cancer that had already spread to her bones and lungs. Although originally the cancer was localized in the breast and very curable, now it was widespread and incurable. Because Mrs. Jones had so little income, we determined that she was eligible for Medicaid, which paid for 100 percent of her tests, medicines, and treatments.

Of course, she had also been eligible for Medicaid even before she developed breast cancer, but regrettably, she never checked with anyone to see what help she could receive. Had she applied for the insurance earlier, before the mass appeared, she would have had a primary-care physician who might have been able to diagnose her breast cancer at an earlier, curable stage. But delaying diagnosis and treatment ultimately cost Mrs. Jones her life.

We always refer to people who are financially challenged, or poor, as "indigent." That word takes on variations of meaning when it comes to health-care access, because, in fact, there are two groups of people who lack resources. First there are the poor—the financially indigent. Government programs exist to create a safety net for them. But then there are the medically indigent, those who lack access to affordable insurance programs. Where is their safety net? What can be done to help them?

## The Financially Indigent

The financially indigent are those people who do not have enough money to buy life's necessities, including needed medical care or medicines. Because of their poverty, such individuals frequently don't have a stable family life. The major obstacle to their health care is identifying a medical resource (a doctor's office, clinic, or hospital) from which they can get good, reliable, continuing care. When they feel sick, they usually get evaluated at an emergency room.

The government defines financial indigence using the official federal *poverty guideline* (also sometimes called the "federal poverty level"). Published annually in the federal register, this guideline changes each year and is determined by the Department of Health and Human Services. In 2011, the poverty guideline was $10,890 for an individual and $22,350 for a family of four. The guideline is 15 percent higher in Hawaii and 25 percent higher in Alaska. (For the current guideline, visit ASPE.HHS.gov.) Federal assistance programs use the poverty guideline as a criterion for eligibility. Note that the poverty guideline is not the same as the *poverty threshold*, which is defined annually by the Census Bureau in order to develop poverty population figures; the poverty threshold is not used to determine assistance eligibility.

Fortunately, there is a national medical insurance safety net for many financially indigent individuals. This is the Medicaid system. If you have a low income and are in a designated eligibility group, you are probably eligible for Medicaid. (In 2011, Medicaid eligibility was set at a maximum of 133 percent of the federal poverty guideline.) There are seven nationally designated eligibility groups, who must meet poverty guidelines that differ by group, from 100 to 135 percent of the federal poverty level. They are pregnant women; children under nineteen; adults who care for children under eighteen; people on supplemental security income; people under age twenty-one living on their own; blind or disabled individuals; and certain people over age sixty-five. In addition to these federally mandated eligible groups, thirty-four states have defined Medicaid eligibility by poverty level only. For more information, check with your state health department or visit Benefits.gov.

Unless you already have Medicaid insurance, the usual gateways into the Medicaid system are an emergency room, a state health department office, or a social worker. Although these systems may be slow or cumbersome, they are worth the wait to get into the Medicaid plan. Once you have Medicaid, you can schedule visits with a primary-care physician, and testing, treatments, and medications can be prescribed—and it's all paid for by the government health plan.

If you think you might be eligible for Medicaid because of your income, do not wait until you're sick to apply. By delaying your application, you may miss the opportunity to cure a condition in its treatable stages. My patient Mrs. Jones died because of that delay. Do not let her story become yours.

## The Medically Indigent

So who are the medically indigent? These are people who do not have health insurance and cannot pay for large medical bills, but who have too many resources to be eligible for Medicaid. Too poor to afford insurance, too "rich" to get Medicaid, these individuals simply fall through the cracks in our health-care system.

For example, I know a woman who worked intermittently in the movie industry. She felt she could not afford private health insurance, but she had too many assets and too high an income to be eligible for Medicaid. When she developed blood in her urine, an expensive emergency-room visit found a lump on her kidney. Without insurance, she had to pay cash for a private consultation with a urologist, and she then paid a negotiated discounted rate at a hospital to have the mass removed. She was cured, but only after accumulating a large medical debt because she had allowed herself to become medically indigent. As a result, she was pushed to the brink of bankruptcy.

But she could have avoided that scenario. By choosing a very high-deductible health plan, she could have had almost all her debt covered by insurance after an affordable deductible. She could have paid out of pocket to have minor problems treated at an urgent-care office (usually situated in pharmacies or in stand-alone buildings, they are much less expensive than emergency rooms). She could have paid for doctors' visits once or twice a year for preventive care. Then, when she needed the expensive hospital stay, the insurance coverage would have kicked in after the first few thousand dollars (which she could have put on her credit card and paid off over time).

There are other ways to access care. Go to your local hospital and talk to a social worker to see if there are any health plans that could help you to get care at the hospital if you need it. Sometimes the social worker will know of charity funds that may be available to help you in case of a catastrophic injury or illness. Your city or county may have a clinic available to help in your care, and social workers can help enroll you. Community health clinics can provide good care if you have no insurance and limited financial resources, even if you lack Medicaid. And social workers there can help you apply for insurance like Medicaid if you are eligible, and they can guide you in obtaining information, forms, and support.

Consider finding a new job that offers health care, even if the insurance plan is only of fair quality. Having insurance can be the difference between life and death if you are suddenly struck by a disease or illness.

Whether or not you have health insurance, if you become ill, immediately see a doctor or get to an emergency room to get the care you need. Worry about the bills later, after you have gotten the care to keep you healthy. Use the city or county health-care system, if necessary.

## Tips

- If you are poor and lack health insurance, apply for Medicaid. You probably qualify.
- If you are uninsured and have a low or moderate income, read the chapter on shopping for insurance and consider a high-deductible catastrophic insurance plan. Talk to an insurance broker for advice.
- If you lack insurance due to prior poor health or a diagnosed condition, consider a state-administered high-risk pool that may make insurance available to you.

- Even if you are medically or financially poor, be certain that you have a primary doctor. Doctors can be affordable, and some will even give you a discount for paying with cash or by credit card.

## Modern Medicine and the Medically Underserved

Since a major effort in health-care reform is to enable society to meet the needs of people without health insurance, new and improved programs for the medically underserved are appearing every year. Keep up with these changes. In 2010, the Patient Protection and Affordable Care Act increased funding for community health centers, increased the number of community health workers, and increased the number of patients they serve. The act has created community-based collaborative health networks and health teams (promoting "medical homes" for patients). And by seeking to reduce cultural barriers to access, it has made health care more available to people who would otherwise have difficulty getting it.

The results of these national, state, and local changes have been to make more resources available for obtaining care. So check with your city, county, and state health departments to see what kind of care is available to you. Take advantage of those resources, even if you're not sick. And if you can't find any resources today, check back in two or three months to see if a new program has begun.

# Chapter 30

# Finding Affordable Medications

It astonishes patients how expensive prescriptions have become. Our remarkably more effective drugs also have remarkably high prices. That creates stress and, often, noncompliance with physician treatment plans, just to save money. How can you deal with this expensive component of health care?

## The History of Effective Drugs

Pharmaceuticals have dramatically impacted the lives of every American. From the beginning to the end of the twentieth century, the average lifespan for Americans nearly doubled. Chemicals and medicines enabled them to live to see not just their grandchildren, but also their great-grandchildren. Pesticides controlled diseases like yellow fever and malaria. Chemical water purification eradicated cholera and dysentery. Potent antibiotics cured fatal pneumonias and serious infections. Vaccinations prevented many conditions, from measles to polio. Antihypertensive blood pressure drugs brought debilitating and potentially fatal strokes and heart attacks under control. Over the course of a single century, medicine was able, through research, clinical trials, and the development of our medical delivery system, to give added life to every person in the United States. The drug industry has proven its worth to mankind.

Medication has proven its value not only in length of life, but also in quality of life. Such valuable drugs as antidepressants, antianxiety medications, and antipsychotics now allow patients formerly incapacitated by mental illness to live productive, happy lives with their families. Extended-release narcotics, antiarthritis steroidal and nonsteroidal anti-inflammatory medications, and transdermal opiate drug patches enable patients previously bedridden with pain to now enjoy themselves. Osteoporosis is controlled with estrogens and bisphosphonates, while high cholesterol is effectively treated with cholesterol-lowering statins. Even many cancers are now preventable with well-tolerated medications such as tamoxifen, raloxifene, and aromatase inhibitors (breast cancer); aspirin and celecoxib (colon cancer); and finasteride and statins (prostate cancer).

But because our life span has increased, chronic diseases are now more prevalent, along with the need for more medicines to control them. And each time a more potent drug is discovered, its cost is higher than that of the medicine used before. As a result, the family drug bill has grown higher. Many elderly patients, who often live on fixed incomes, now are having to decide whether to buy the medicines they need or pay their rent and food bills.

## Pharmaceutical Insurance Coverage

Many insurance plans have a pharmaceutical drug benefit. HMOs typically have at least some drug benefit, but the drug formulary (the list of drugs covered for payment) may be limited. The Veterans Administration provides a wide range of medications to veterans. (If you are a veteran, you can get more information by calling 800-827-1000.) Medicaid usually covers some or all the expense of medically necessary drugs, especially if they are generic. PPO health plans also frequently have drug benefits.

While Medicare did not have a prescription drug benefit in the past, the Medicare Modernization Act passed in 2003 made optional drug coverage available. This is known as Medicare Part D. Under this provision, if your income is low you can receive drug coverage for free. If you do not qualify for free drugs because your income is higher, you will have to pay for your Part D coverage, choosing among the competing plans in your area. Factors like cost, deductibles, and co-payments vary among plans, and they can change every year. As you choose a plan, here are the typical variables to consider as of 2012:

- **Deductible:** You may pay 100 percent of the first $320 of your drug costs, or you may pay nothing—this varies from plan to plan.
- **Initial benefit period:** For the next $2,610 or so of your drug costs, you may pay only 25 percent ($500), but again, this varies among plans.
- **The doughnut hole (or gap in coverage):** For the next $3,727 of your drug costs, you may pay 100 percent, but this varies among plans and may be discounted if you use more expensive proprietary drugs. Also, the Patient Protection and Affordable Care Act reduces what you must pay: for brand name drugs, you pay only 50 percent of the cost (decreasing to 25 percent by 2020) and for generic drugs, you pay only 86 percent of the cost (decreasing to 25 percent by 2020).
- **Second benefit period:** For all subsequent drug costs, you may pay only 5 percent of whatever the medicines cost.

In addition, some companies offer more than one Part D plan, and those plans vary in terms of which medicines are covered, how much they charge for each medicine, what co-pay they require, and what other help they will give you in managing your drug treatments. So you will have to do some fancy comparative shopping. If you have a limited income, the Medicare "Extra Help" program further discounts medication costs.

Now, since that is very complicated, you must carefully evaluate your drug expenses to see if a particular benefit will actually help you lower your overall medication costs. For more information, as well as an Internet tool to help you compare each of the various plans available in your community under Medicare Part D, visit Medicare.gov and look under "Medicare prescription drug coverage." You can also turn to your local pharmacy for help, as every pharmacist is now working with patients to provide guidance about the least expensive way to access Medicare Part D coverage. Your health-insurance broker is another good resource as you decide which Part D plan is best for you.

Be certain to check your health plan to determine the extent of your drug coverage, any deductible or exclusions, any preauthorization requirements, and whether generic drugs and proprietary drugs are paid for equally.

There are many federal and state programs that offer prescription discounts, including state pharmaceutical assistance programs (SPAPs). To check out eligibility requirements for these programs, or to evaluate the applicability of pharmaceutical company discount programs, visit BenefitsCheckup. org.

## Receiving Your Initial Prescription

Generic drugs (which are no longer restricted by a patent, and which are manufactured by several companies) are much less expensive than proprietary drugs (drugs still protected by a patent and made by only one company). If your doctor is prescribing a new medicine, you should always ask, "**Is there a generic version of this drug**, or is another generic drug just as good?" This may save you a lot of money.

Sometimes there is an over-the-counter medicine that's just as effective as the medication for which your doctor was going to write a prescription. So your next question should be, "**Is there an over-the-counter medicine that is cheaper and just as good as the prescription?**"

Next, you should know that many drugs come in different strengths, and often it is possible to **buy a double-strength pill and cut it in half** using an inexpensive pill-splitter you can purchase in any pharmacy. Not all pills can be split, however, and *no* capsules can be split. Ask your pharmacist or physician if it would be safe and save you money to use this method, since it might reduce your cost by as much as half.

You can also ask if the doctor has **free samples** of the new medicine. Not only will free doses lower your initial costs, but they also will save you money if you have a bad reaction to the drug and have to stop taking it. (Otherwise, if you have already bought a one-month supply of the drug, twenty-five to thirty days' worth may have to be discarded.)

Many drug companies offer discounted or even free medications for patients with a limited income (although the criteria for that vary from company to company). But you won't get enrolled in such a program automatically. If you want to get **free or very discounted medicine from the manufacturer**, you will have to ask your doctor, nurse, or pharmacist, or call the company that makes the medicine. (Find the phone number on the drug company website.) The *Physicians' Desk Reference* and its website, PDR.net, list the phone numbers of the manufacturer of every medicine, making it easy to call any drug company's patient information line. But if you don't have access to that resource, just ask your pharmacist. Anytime your doctor prescribes a new medicine for you, ask him if there is a discount program through the manufacturer. He also may have rebate or discount coupon, so ask if one is available. If he doesn't know, go to the manufacturer's website to find out.

If you are receiving very expensive medication, such as oncology chemotherapy drugs, you may have very high co-payments or drug costs, even reaching into the thousands of dollars. Some drug companies donate money to foundations that help patients pay the cost or co-payment for these expensive drugs. These foundations frequently run out of money before the end of the year, however, so apply for these funds as soon as you experience high out-of-pocket expense for your costly prescription medications.

## Comparison Shopping for Price

Comparison shopping for prescription medications isn't always easy, and it can be tedious. To get the lowest price and limit your drug expenses, you must put in some effort to contact the many retailers of medications.

- Start at **your neighborhood pharmacy or the pharmacy in your doctor's office building**. These pharmacies are convenient and can provide a range of services, often including home delivery, as well as information and guidance. Ask if they will meet the best price you can find elsewhere, which they often will agree to do.
- **Discount stores** often have pharmacies that can offer lower-priced medicine, especially on generic drugs. Comparison shop at each of these stores, at least by phone or website; to get the best discount, check their websites as well as their store prices. When I shop for my own medicine, I always include Costco, Walmart, and Target to compare prices for the same drug.

AARP also offers pharmacy services to its members (those over fifty years old) through a network of retail pharmacies nationwide. To find a participating pharmacy near you, visit AARPPharmacy.com.

- **Internet pharmacies** offer prescriptions by mail. Go to Google or another search engine, type in "internet pharmacies," and you will find a complete list, which will likely include Costco. com, CVS.com, and Drugstore.com. If you plan to use an Internet pharmacy, check out the pros and cons as well as a list of disreputable sources at the Food and Drug Administration website, FDA.gov. To see price comparisons for various online pharmacies, visit PharmacyChecker.com. Online pharmacies are often less expensive for certain drugs, but one of your local pharmacies may match their price on many medicines. So when researching Internet pricing, remember to compare prices with those you can obtain locally through a discount store, or—if you're considering a foreign supplier—through American online pharmacies. Compare not only price, but also services provided.

  To see if a particular Internet pharmacy or discount local pharmacy is licensed, check the website of the National Association of Boards of Pharmacies at NABP.net.

- If you are a veteran, the **VA system** offers very low-cost drugs, so be sure to check with your local VA office about the benefits available to you.

## International Purchasing

Among the most popular ways to get discount medication is through Canada or Mexico. Many drugs are less expensive this way, but surprisingly, some medicine can actually be obtained just as inexpensively in the United States.

At the time of publication of this book, importing American-manufactured medications from other countries was illegal. According to our government, this is because the FDA cannot certify the safety, effectiveness, and reliable production of drugs that are imported, as they may have been adulterated, tampered with, or allowed to expire. However, the FDA has a discretionary policy regarding the importation of prescription drugs.

Under the guidelines "Coverage of Personal Importation," the FDA and Customs can use discretion in whether or not to seize drugs you are importing, depending on four criteria. Usually, drugs will *not* be seized by Customs if …

- the FDA has not approved the drug for use, but your use is for a serious condition for which treatment in the United States may be unavailable;
- there is no commercialization of the drug by a distributor;
- your use of the drug does not represent an unreasonable risk;
- you provide a written statement that the drug is for your own use, that it is less than a three-month supply, and that you have a physician in the United States who has prescribed it (or it is the continuation of a treatment started in a foreign country).

Many Americans, including many of my patients, import their drugs from Canada on the Internet. If you do an Internet search for "Canada pharmacies," you will certainly find a long list, which will usually include CanadaMeds.com, Adv-Care.com, RxNorth.com, and CanadianMedService.com. If you are going to pursue this approach—and keep in mind that this is also currently illegal—you must compare prices, as they can vary by up to 20 percent.

Since 2004, some United States drug companies have stopped selling their medicines to certain Canadian pharmacies in order to try to stop this reimportation. In response, some Canadian Internet pharmacies started importing the drugs from countries other than the United States, and then just shipping them back out to patients in the United States. These transshipped medicines are *not inspected* by Canadian authorities and don't have the safeguards and guarantees of Canadian laws and regulations, which are otherwise very good. So if you are using a Canadian Internet pharmacy, be sure to check with it about the source of the drugs you are ordering. If you can't make sure they have not been shipped in from other countries besides the United States, shop elsewhere. The quality of your medicines means everything, so don't accept inferior drugs upon which your life could depend. And anytime you want to use an Internet pharmacy, call its toll-free number to get human answers to critical questions. Ask who the manufacturer is, whether the medicine is produced by an FDA-approved manufacturer, whether the medicine comes in individual unit doses, if the pharmacy undergoes regular quality control checks, if it provides a guarantee of customer satisfaction, and whether customers experience any problems that can be avoided.

Medications are available through other countries as well. For example, lower prices may be available from pharmacies in Israel through IsraMeds.com (phone 866-477-2289). Using this source requires a brief statement of your medical condition, lab tests, a description of current treatments, and a list of other medications being taken, since an Israeli doctor will have to give authorization.

Since importation of American-made drugs violates federal regulations, you must remember that drugs imported in this manner may be subject to confiscation by Customs. In contrast, many states are realizing how much money their own Medicaid programs could save if they purchased their drugs from Canada. As a result, some states are considering legislation permitting importation for use by state programs, which would still potentially conflict with the federal prohibition. To make the current situation even more confusing, there are several bills before Congress that would allow for drug importation by patients. When you read this book, check with US Customs and ask if prescription drug importation is still illegal. You can also check current regulations online at FDA.gov.

If the federal prohibition against drug importation for personal use really angers you, you don't have to just grin and bear it. Write, e-mail, or call your congressman and senators to complain about the effect this rule is having on you. Enlist their support in helping you and others correct the system fairly while retaining the protections against adulterated or imitation drugs, protections which FDA regulations have given us. For the phone number of your legislator, check the "blue pages" of your telephone book, go to your local library, or visit Congress.org.

## Are You Getting Enough Medicine?

With all the medicines many people with chronic diseases are already receiving, "Are you getting enough medicine?" sounds like a foolish question. But in our health-care system today, there is constant pressure from insurers, HMOs, IPAs, and utilization review personnel advising doctors to reduce prescription drug use whenever possible. Ask your own doctor whether you are receiving all the medicine that can possibly help your condition improve, regardless of cost. Has she been pressured not to provide a new medication because of its cost, because she fears insurance company denials, or because she is afraid she will be profiled by the insurance company as a "high-prescribing" physician?

By contrast, have you limited your own use of medicines due to fear of cost? Some patients try to save money by refusing to take a more expensive medicine, even if it will produce better results. I have seen plenty of patients who simply give themselves a drug "holiday" because they want to try to get by without taking pills. Although occasionally this can work, more often the illness worsens as a result—sometimes to the point of hospitalization and severe, irreversible changes.

If you are considering reducing your medications for any reason, always discuss it with your doctor honestly, so he can advise you of the risks involved. Sometimes, faced with your resolve to take fewer medicines, your doctor can suggest alternative therapies to save money or avoid side effects.

## Tips

- When your doctor prescribes medications for you, always take them, regardless of cost. But also talk with him about samples, low-cost programs, and generics.
- If a medication is not making you better, or if you are having a reaction to it, call your physician at once for further instructions. Don't continue to take expensive medicines if they are not working.
- Review all your current medications with your physician at each visit to see if any of them can be stopped, or replaced with cheaper or newer drugs.
- If you can afford it, buy prescription drug insurance. Shop wisely, comparing various plans.
- Always shop for drugs considering both price and pharmacist support services. Don't let price considerations interfere with your health and, ultimately, your own survival.

## Today's Health Care and Medications

Through science and technology, medicine is developing innovative and more effective drugs that can save your life. This is the best of times for scientific achievements; our only problem is how to economically transfer these advances into deliverable treatments in our health-care system. Although health-care reforms are trying to facilitate these improvements, the cost of new medications is still daunting.

Increasingly, the development of molecular and genetic testing will give physicians the ability to know which patients can benefit from a new medicine and which patients can't. Meanwhile, national societies of specialty physicians will continue to develop guidelines about which patients need certain new treatments and which do not. It will become your job to do your own research about advances in treating your illness or condition. Ask your doctor about those new advances and any testing that might indicate if you would benefit from them. The goal is getting the right medicines to the right patients at the right time.

At the same time, health plans and insurers are trying to reduce medication costs. So expect more frequent denials of prescription coverage; you may have to insist on appealing those denials to get insurance coverage for medications you need. Partnering with your doctor will be most important, so have a doctor you trust.

# Epilogue

# Contemporary Medicine and Health-Care Reform: Will You Survive?

With or without reforms and changes, it is becoming more difficult to manage your health care. Insurance and care are more expensive, health-insurance plans are more confusing, communicating with your doctor and his or her office is more cumbersome—and you are always left wondering if you're getting all the treatments and preventive care you need.

With the passage of the Patient Protection and Affordable Care Act and its approval by the Supreme Court, Americans will have more protections in their health insurance, but also more likelihood that their insurance rules and regulations will change. Some people will loose their health benefits from their employers. To complicate matters further, the executive branch will write thousands of pages of new regulations, which will change how insurance functions. Congress will likely further amend (or even repeal) the act. So you have more responsibility to keep informed of changes in your insurance (your doctor, employer, insurance agent and/or the Medicare website will be your best resources).

The chapters in this book have addressed the most important aspects of health care and provided suggestions and tools to help you. And keep in mind that no matter what changes evolve in our health-care system, certain basic principles will remain.

## Basic Principles

- Choose the best insurance you can afford.
- Choose the best primary doctor and specialists appropriate to your illnesses who are affiliated with your insurance.
- Choose the best hospital covered by your insurance.
- Use the Internet to get information about your illnesses and disease prevention, and review this information with your physician.
- Get a second opinion using the guidelines I have suggested.
- Keep your own medical record and take a copy of that record to your appointments and hospitalizations.
- Take a written list of questions to your appointments, and bring home written notes from your visit. Have an advocate to help you. Since doctor visits will be shorter, go over your questions or problems efficiently but completely.
- Do not become frustrated or discouraged with your illness or with the medical-care system. Follow your doctor's advice, or find a doctor whose advice you will follow.
- Expect changes in your insurance, covered benefits, contracted physicians, and costs of care, and use the advice in this book to handle those changes.

Your survival depends on your taking increased responsibility for your care. It may take a lot of time and persistence, but your reward will be greater confidence, more trust in your health-care team, better health, and a longer, happier life.

So there you have it: the advice I give my patients, my family, and my friends. Now it is up to you to make a choice. Will you use your intelligence and judgment to make good decisions … and survive? Or despite all the changes in modern medicine and continuing health-care reforms, will you go through life as you have before … and suffer more illness, disability, and possible premature demise by being unprepared? Life or death—the choice is in your hands. Now you have the power to choose life.

# About the Author

Writing authoritatively about a comprehensive approach to getting better health care requires an author with extensive and varied experience in patient care and administration. Dr. Cary Presant, board certified in internal medicine and hematology, has spent more than forty years caring for patients. Initially this was in academic medicine at university hospitals, including Columbia University, the National Institutes of Health and National Cancer Institute, Washington University School of Medicine, City of Hope National Medical Center, and the University of Southern California Keck School of Medicine. He was the director of medical oncology at City of Hope and is professor of clinical medicine at the University of Southern California.

Next Dr. Presant developed clinical programs in community cancer centers and hospitals. He was the chairman of the Los Angeles Cancer Institute at St. Vincent's Medical Center in Los Angeles and headed cancer programs in Queen of the Valley Hospital, Intercommunity Hospital, and Citrus Valley Health Partners in the San Gabriel Valley section of Los Angeles.

Always seeking better care for his patients, Dr. Presant has conducted research throughout his career. Author of more than four hundred scientific articles, book chapters, and other publications, he has concentrated on new drug development, combination drug therapy for many different cancers, the use of liposomes (microscopic fat bubbles) to make chemotherapy more active and less toxic, quality-of-life measurement in cancer patients, and development of laboratory tests to personalize cancer therapy. He invented a new drug, DaunoXome, and he helped develop a drug company, Vestar

Pharmaceuticals, which has produced anticancer drugs and antibiotics. Presently he is also the chief medical officer at DiaTech Oncology, which tests apoptosis induced by drugs to determine drug sensitivity of cancers.

As an administrator, Dr. Presant was principle investigator of the Central Los Angeles Community Clinical Oncology Program and president of the California Cancer Medical Center. He led national medical organizations, becoming a director of the American Society of Clinical Oncology, president of the Association of Community Cancer Centers, and president and chairman of the Medical Oncology Association of Southern California. In those positions, he has worked with congressmen, senators, White House administrators, and California legislators to help formulate health-care policy.

In his work with nonprofit health-care organizations, he has served as president of the American Cancer Society California Division and has been on the board of directors of the health-care advocacy group Cancer Schmancer. As a medical writer, Dr. Presant has been a columnist for Medscape.com, where he now publishes a blog on cancer health care.

With his experience in medical practice, research, academic centers, community care, health-care reform, and patient advocacy, Dr. Presant is the expert who can address the many and complex issues covered in this book from the perspectives of the patient, the doctor, and the health-care system.

# Appendixes

# Appendix 1

# An Outline for Your Personal Medical Record

## 1. Demographics

Name, address, date of birth, height, Social Security number, driver's license number, home phone, pager, mobile phone, fax, e-mail, employer, work phone; emergency contact name(s), address, home phone, work phone, pager, mobile phone, fax, e-mail; your religion; spouse or significant other's name and phone number; children's names and phone numbers. Add durable power of attorney for health care form, if you have signed one.

Optional: Name, address, and phone number of lawyer, accountant, and clergy.

Optional: If you are keeping a personal medical record, include a list of any other people who have a copy of it, along with their with name, address, e-mail, phone number, and cell phone number.

## 2. Insurance

Fill out information for each company through which you have health insurance, and keep a photocopy of the front and back of each insurance card. Include the name of the company, name of insured, certificate number, group number, effective date, and phone numbers for the company and for preauthorization.

## 3. Problem List

List each of your medical problems separately, including a brief description of the problem and its severity and date of onset; its response to treatments; its evolution (whether it's getting better or worse); any association with diet, activity, or medicines; prior occurrences of the problem; and the date the problem resolved, if applicable.

## 4. Your Doctors and Health-Care Team

List separately each of your current physicians as well as any physicians you have seen in the past.

Primary-care doctor: Note whether current or past (and date); address, phone number, fax, e-mail, and website; names of nurses, administrator, billing person, and covering doctors; and the phone number of the answering service.

Consultants: Same information as above.

Hospital(s): Note whether current or past, including dates of admission (if any) and address, phone number, and fax number. For the current hospital, also include nurses' names on each floor you have used and extension number (if appropriate); contact name and number for patient advocacy office; and name of president or chief executive officer (for sending thanks or complaints, or for praising individual staff members).

Social worker

Dietician

Psychologist

Rehabilitation program

Laboratory used

Radiology departments used

Others on health care team

## 5. Medication Record

List all prescription drugs and vitamins taken, including over-the-counter drugs. For each medication, list the following: name; dose; reason for taking medicine; dates started and stopped; any reaction or allergy; pharmacy name, phone number, and address; prescription number; and name of pharmacist.

## 6. Allergies or Intolerance to Drugs

Note medicine, date of use, and type of reaction.

## 7. Medical History

For each illness or chronic condition, list the following: diagnosis, date condition began or was diagnosed, name and phone number of treating physician, treatment, and date the condition resolved (if applicable).

For each surgery, list the following: diagnosis, type of surgery, date, hospital, surgeon, and any complications.

For each abnormal test, list the following: test, date, and result.

For each functional or psychological change, list the following: symptom, date it began, treatment, treating doctor, and date it resolved (if applicable).

For each change in interpersonal relationships, list the change and date.

For each exposure to toxins (asbestos, benzene, chemicals, radiation, lead, others), list the following: type of exposure, dates the exposure started and stopped, and the situation in which it occurred (at work, including type of work, at home, etc.).

## 8. Family History (see sample form, appendix 2)

## 9. Vaccinations

Note all vaccines, dates given, and any negative reactions.

## 10. Copies of Histories or Reports

Include surgical notes, pathology reports, history and physical reports, consultation notes, discharge summaries, and letters from your doctor to other doctors.

## 11. Copies of Test Reports

Include all laboratory results, X-ray reports, and disease-screening tests.

## 12. Copies of Actual X-Rays

If you have had a serious illness or disease, obtain a copy of any important X-ray (such as an abnormal mammogram, chest X-ray, or CAT scan) for your personal medical record. If you are moving to another city, take all your old X-rays (or copies of them on CD) with you.

## 13. Calendar of Annual Disease-Screening Tests

Include the date you are scheduled to repeat any test.

# 14. Social History

Do you smoke now? Did you smoke in the past? If so, how many packs and for how many years?

Do you now or have you ever used snuff or chewing tobacco?

Do you drink alcohol? Did you drink in the past? If so, what type of alcohol and how much per day?

Have you ever used illicit drugs? If so, which ones and when?

Where were you born? What is your occupation? Do you still work? Have you been exposed to asbestos, radiation or toxic chemicals?

With whom do you live? What do you enjoy doing? What are your hobbies?

Are you or were you married? Is your spouse healthy?

Did (or do) your parents or spouse smoke?

What is your sexual orientation?

**For your current visit with the physician:**

## 1. Question List

Write a list of questions to ask the doctor. Include copies of any newspaper or magazine articles or Internet information you want to discuss.

## 2. Review of Systems (see appendix 3)

Include the form your doctor uses, or use the sample form in appendix 3. Fill it out for each doctor visit.

# Appendix 2

## Sample Family-History Form

Place a check in each box where there has been a disease diagnosed.

For any disease in any family member, write in the space below the specific disease (for example, type of cancer) and the approximate age at which it occurred.

| Name | Relationship | Disease | Age Started |
| --- | --- | --- | --- |

| | Mother | Father | Mother's family | Grandmother | Grandfather |
|---|---|---|---|---|---|
| Hepatitis | | | | | |
| Asthma | | | | | |
| Tuberculosis | | | | | |
| Eye Disease | | | | | |
| Suicide | | | | | |
| Alcoholism | | | | | |
| Depression | | | | | |
| Nervous Disorder | | | | | |
| Stroke | | | | | |
| Muscle Disease | | | | | |
| Cysts (liver, kidney, ovary) | | | | | |
| Lung Disease | | | | | |
| Kidney Disease | | | | | |
| Colitis | | | | | |
| High Blood Pressure | | | | | |
| Heart Disease | | | | | |
| Colon Polyps | | | | | |
| Diabetes | | | | | |
| Anemia | | | | | |
| Bleeding Disorder | | | | | |
| Blood Clots | | | | | |
| Cancer | | | | | |

| | Aunts, uncles (list only those with disease) | Father's family | Grandmother | Grandfather | Aunts, uncles (list only those with disease) |
|---|---|---|---|---|---|
| Hepatitis | | | | | |
| Asthma | | | | | |
| Tuberculosis | | | | | |
| Eye Disease | | | | | |
| Suicide | | | | | |
| Alcoholism | | | | | |
| Depression | | | | | |
| Nervous Disorder | | | | | |
| Stroke | | | | | |
| Muscle Disease | | | | | |
| Cysts (liver, kidney, ovary) | | | | | |
| Lung Disease | | | | | |
| Kidney Disease | | | | | |
| Colitis | | | | | |
| High Blood Pressure | | | | | |
| Heart Disease | | | | | |
| Colon Polyps | | | | | |
| Diabetes | | | | | |
| Anemia | | | | | |
| Bleeding Disorder | | | | | |
| Blood Clots | | | | | |
| Cancer | | | | | |

| | Sisters (list all) | Brothers (list all) | Children (list all) |
|---|---|---|---|
| Hepatitis | | | |
| Asthma | | | |
| Tuberculosis | | | |
| Eye Disease | | | |
| Suicide | | | |
| Alcoholism | | | |
| Depression | | | |
| Nervous Disorder | | | |
| Stroke | | | |
| Muscle Disease | | | |
| Cysts (liver, kidney, ovary) | | | |
| Lung Disease | | | |
| Kidney Disease | | | |
| Colitis | | | |
| High Blood Pressure | | | |
| Heart Disease | | | |
| Colon Polyps | | | |
| Diabetes | | | |
| Anemia | | | |
| Bleeding Disorder | | | |
| Blood Clots | | | |
| Cancer | | | |

# Appendix 3

# Sample Review of Systems

**(Circle areas of concern.)**

**Constitutional:** fever, weight loss, fatigue, night sweats, hot flashes, weakness, pain

**Eyes:** cataracts, decreased vision, irritation of eyes, red eyes

**Ears:** change in hearing, discharge from ears, earache

**Nose:** nasal drainage, nosebleed, stuffy nose, sinus infection, sinus pain

**Mouth:** change in teeth, sore mouth, mouth ulcers, change in sense of taste

**Throat:** sore throat, difficulty swallowing, dryness

**Cardiovascular:** palpitations, chest pain, chest pressure, high blood pressure, low blood pressure, heart disease, heart attacks

**Respiratory:** cough, shortness of breath, wheezing, coughing blood, pneumonia, bronchitis, asthma

**Gastrointestinal:** blood in stool, change in appetite, nausea, vomiting, diarrhea, constipation, bleeding from rectum, hemorrhoids, heartburn, gastritis, GERD, ulcers, polyps, colitis, loss of bowel control, cramps

**Genitourinary:** urinary tract infections, urinating during the night, blood in urine, painful or difficult urination, loss of bladder control, problems with sexual function, change in sex drive, difficulties with intercourse. For women: vaginal dryness, vaginal discharge. For men: problems with erections.

**Musculoskeletal:** leg pain or weakness, bluish discoloration of skin, swelling, joint pain, arthritis, swelling in the joints, fractures, joint replacement, muscle tenderness, muscle weakness

**Skin:** rash, bleeding, tenderness, redness, lacerations, lumps, itching, new moles or masses, change in color or shape or size of mole

**Breasts:** breast pain, redness, lump, swelling, nipple discharge

**Neurologic:** change in thinking, confusion, incoordination, seizures, strokes, weakness of arms, weakness of legs, numbness of arms, numbness of legs, dizziness

**Psychiatric:** anxiety, depression, psychosis, nervousness

**Endocrine:** diabetes, thyroid disorders

**Hematologic/Lymphatic:** anemia, bleeding, swollen lymph nodes, swollen glands, bruising, abnormal blood counts

**Allergic:** allergies, hay fever, frequent infections

**Infections:** repeated infections, tuberculosis (TB), exposure to tuberculosis

Pain Assessment Scale **(Circle the number that best describes your pain.)**

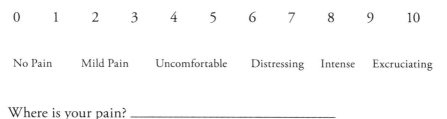

| 0 | 1 | 2 | 3 | 4 | 5 | 6 | 7 | 8 | 9 | 10 |
|---|---|---|---|---|---|---|---|---|---|----|

No Pain    Mild Pain    Uncomfortable    Distressing    Intense    Excruciating

Where is your pain? _____

What is the nature of the pain? _____

## Energy Scale (How much energy or strength do you have?)

0    10%   20%   30%   40%   50%   60%   70%   80%   90%   100%

No Strength                                           Normal Strength

## Quality-of-Life Scale (What is your quality of life?)

0     1     2     3     4     5     6     7     8     9     10

Very Poor   Poor         Adequate    Good         Very Good   Excellent

**Have you seen any new physicians since your last visit? If so, whom?**

**Have you been in the emergency room or hospital since your last visit? If so, where?**

**Have you traveled outside this city since your last visit? If so, where?**

**Have you started any new medications since your last visit? If so, which ones? Are they prescription, or over-the-counter?**

**Have you had any operations or biopsies since your last visit? If so, explain.**

**Have you had any tests or X-rays since your last visit? If so, note the nature of any test or X-ray and when it was done.**

# Appendix 4

# State Medical Board and Insurance Commissioner Contacts

**State Medical Boards and Osteopathic Boards:** Some states have separate medical and osteopathic boards, and some states have only one. To contact the board(s) in any state, visit the website of the Federation of State Medical boards, FSMB.org, and click on "Contact a State Medical Board." You will see the website address, phone number, and fax number for each board and the name of its executive director.

**State Insurance Commissioners:** To contact the insurance commissioner in any state, visit the website of the National Association of Insurance Commissioners, NAIC.org. You will see the name and photograph of the commissioner, and the physical address, phone and fax numbers, and website address for the commissioner's office.

# Appendix 5

# Sample Letter to Insurance Appealing a Denial

**Insurance company name**
**Insurance company address**
**c/o Appeals Office**
**RE: Insert Your insurance policy number and your date of birth**
**Dear Madam or Sir:**

I am writing to appeal your denial of a request for authorization (or claim for payment for services) dated _____. This was submitted by my physician, Dr. _____. The service requested (or performed) was _____ for my illness _____. I was assured by my physician that this was medically necessary and the standard of care for my illness. Without this I will suffer illness or injury or damage to my body as follows: _____.

I believe your denial was inappropriate, and I request that you approve the request for authorization (or payment for the claim). If you feel that you will again deny approval, I ask that you use a reviewer who is a medical specialist in my disease and advise me of the name of the reviewer. I am very concerned about my health and do not wish to have my condition worsen, so I ask that you review and approve the request as soon as possible without delay.

Thank you for your prompt assistance and action.

Sincerely
Your name

CC:

**Medical Director of Insurance Company (put his or her name here; you can get it from the insurance company information line.)**
**State Insurance Commissioner (you can get his or her name and address using resources in appendix 4.)**